THE HAPPINESS EFFECT

OTHER TITLES BY EARL MINDELL RPh, MH, PhD

Earl Mindell's Allergy Bible

Earl Mindell's Anti-Aging Bible

Earl Mindell's Food As Medicine

Dr. Earl Mindell's Memory Bible

Earl Mindell's New Herb Bible

Earl Mindell's Supplement Bible

Dr. Earl Mindell's Vitamin D Miracle

Prescription Alternatives, 4th Edition
with Virginia Hopkins, MA

Dr. Earl Mindell's The Power of MSM
with Virginia Hopkins, MA

Earl Mindell's New Vitamin Bible, 6th Edition
with Hester Mundis

THE HAPPINESS EFFECT

THE POSITIVE BENEFITS OF NEGATIVE IONS

Earl Mindell, RPh, MH, PhD

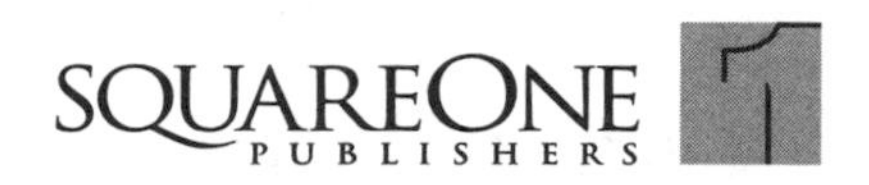

The information and advice contained in this book are based upon the research and the personal and professional experiences of the author. They are not intended as a substitute for consulting with a health care professional. The publisher and author are not responsible for any adverse effects or consequences resulting from the use of any of the suggestions, preparations, or procedures discussed in this book. All matters pertaining to your physical health should be supervised by a health care professional. It is a sign of wisdom, not cowardice, to seek a second or third opinion.

Cover Designer: Jeannie Tudor
Editor: Michael Weatherhead
Typesetter: Gary A. Rosenberg

Square One Publishers
115 Herricks Road
Garden City Park, NY 11040
(877) 900-BOOK
www.squareonepublishers.com

Library of Congress Cataloging-in-Publication Data

Names: Mindell, Earl.
Title: The happiness effect / Earl Mindell.
Description: Garden City Park, NY : Square One Publishers, [2016] | Includes bibliographical references and index.
Identifiers:LCCN 2015034039 | ISBN 9780757004223 (paper)
ISBN 9780757054228 (ebook)
Subjects: LCSH: Naturopathy. | Anions. | Ions—Physiological effect.
Classification: LCC RZ605 .M56 2016 | DDC 615.5/35—dc23 LC record available at http://lccn.loc.gov/2015034039

Photo on page 21 courtesy of Patricia Sisler.

Printed in the United States of America

10 9 8 7 6 5 4 3 2 1

Contents

To my wonderful, beautiful, and talented grandchildren, Lily and Ryan.
Thank you for having a "happiness effect" on our family every day.

Acknowledgments

No truly comprehensive text such as this one is ever the work of just one person. Over the course of writing this book, helpful contributions came from a number of different sources, leaving me with many people to thank. I would first like to thank Patricia Sisler, daughter of Dr. Clarence Hansell, for the background information on her father and his pioneering work in the field of negative ions. Without Dr. Hansell's dogged perseverance in the face of an unknown phenomenon he felt deserving of study, the power of negative ions might have been left unexamined, and this book certainly would not have been written. Patricia supplied me with the documentation I required to shed light on her father's important work. I am lucky to have been able to find her, and I am grateful that she was so responsive to my requests.

I would like to thank my editor, Michael Weatherhead, who essentially took the rough draft I'd given him and crafted it into a readable, intelligible, and thorough book. His keen sense of structure and highly skeptical eye kept me on track and set this work on a solid foundation. Such critical resolve was necessary to bring credibility to this incredible subject.

Special thanks go to my publisher, Rudy Shur, who had the open mind and generous spirit to get behind this project and see it through to its best possible conclusion. It goes without saying that I could not have done this without him, but I will continue to say it anyway.

Lastly, it is absolutely imperative that I thank the many scientists and researchers who, over the past handful of decades, have taken the time to conduct and publish studies on negative ions and their effects. The field of negative ions has been one of little interest to the mainstream medical establishment up to this point, and performing good research on this subject is not in any way considered a means of achieving notoriety or earning praise. It is a thankless job at the moment, which is part of the reason I have written this book. I hope its publication moves the subject of negative ions from the fringe of the medical world to a place of acceptance.

Preface

As a registered pharmacist, I have always found it ironic that so many doctors view the use of nutrition to heal the body as some sort of alternative medicine. In spite of the fact that countless studies have demonstrated the protective effects of good nutrition, our medical system is rooted in the belief that medication is the only means of relief from our most common health ailments. In an effort to change this mindset, I have spent over thirty years of my life writing books on the topic of nutrition and health, so I was surprised to find myself writing a different type of health book recently. I hadn't really planned on writing this book, but sometimes something catches your attention, and you just have to go with your gut. So, why write a book on negative ions? You can thank billionaire Mark Cuban.

As it turns out, one of the shows my wife and I enjoy watching is *Shark Tank*. It's a clever show on which entrepreneurs of start-up companies are given a few minutes to pitch their products or ideas in front of a group of potential investors, or "sharks," as they like to be called. Once a pitch is over, the "sharks" are given an opportunity to question the presenter. Understandably, these investors often want to know how far the entrepreneur has gone with the idea, how much money the business has made, what the presenter's business background is, and what the future may hold for the business. Once the questions end, each "shark" has an opportunity to make a cash bid for a percentage of the business. The premise is simple and the results can be life-changing for the contestant. On one particular occasion, however, something happened that just didn't seem right—at least it didn't seem right in my opinion.

A young man was introduced as having a wristband that reversed certain health issues. It was based on the fact that the band emitted negative ions. As he began his pitch, Mark Cuban, one of the investors on the panel, interrupted him to ask what the science was behind the product. The young man looked at Mark like a deer caught in the headlights. Mark asked him again. Whether or not the man had an answer, by the look on his face, it was evident that he was not prepared to respond to such a question, or that he was simply in a state of shock—which I'm assuming could happen when you are being recorded for television. The second non-response was the beginning of Mark's tirade against the product. Cuban boiled the whole thing down to quackery. Needless to say, that pretty much ended the presenter's pitch as well as his chances of getting any "shark" to back his product.

Over the next day or two, I thought about that segment and the way in which the product was dismissed outright as worthless. Now, while I didn't know a great deal about negative ions at the time, I knew several people who had worn similar bracelets, and who had told me how they had worked for them. Out of curiosity, I began to read up on the topic. Through an online search, I found there were hundreds of websites devoted to the negative ions. I began reading everything I came across, and, as is my habit, I started taking notes. What I found was very interesting. There were sites that provided scientific studies on the benefits of negative ions, sites that sold negative-ion products with their own takes on the associated health benefits, and sites that called negative-ion products all a big sham. It was, however, the abundance of positive scientific research that won me over. But if what I was reading was true, why hadn't the many health benefits of negative ions become common knowledge instead of holding the dishonorable title of quack medicine?

Over the course of the next few months, I began to do more and more research on this subject. It became clear to me that there was, indeed, a jumble of fact and fiction running wild on the Internet. I began, slowly but surely, to sort out the truth. Where a so-called fact or study was cited, if I could not find its original source, I would eliminate it from consideration. Additionally, as I began to put the pieces together, I learned of the fascinating history behind the development and use of negative ions. This history also pointed out how the medicinal establishment of the 1950s, 1960s, and 1970s—to put it kindly—minimized the health benefits of negative ions. By the time my work was done, I realized I had enough to put together a book on the topic—a book that would, perhaps, answer Mark Cuban's question, "Where's the science?"

In closing, let me make the following points: I believe what you will find as you read *The Happiness Effect* is a simple and economic way to mitigate a number of health issues with absolutely no side effects. I believe negative ions may work better for some individuals than others due to biochemical differences between our bodies, but I also believe negative ions can be a blessing to many people. I will also say that, as a consumer, you must always make certain the product you wish to purchase is up to par. While I have provided some guidelines regarding negative-ion devices in this book, you should always do your homework before buying any product that may affect your health. I hope you find this book helpful.

Be well,

Dr. Earl Mindell, RPh, MH, PhD
Beverly Hills, California

Introduction

What if I were to tell you there is a force found in nature that can provide you with a feeling of well-being, energize you, allow you to sleep better, relieve your allergies, increase your ability to concentrate, and cheer you up? Sounds crazy, right? But this force exists, and it's something that you cannot get from a bottle of prescription drugs.

While the pharmaceutical industry certainly has a wide variety of pills to offer those afflicted with health conditions, the problem is that most of these options are expensive and associated with potentially dangerous side effects. While millions, if not billions, of dollars have been spent in the marketing of these problematic options, there has been a simple, natural, low-cost remedy available that may be beneficial in the treatment of a handful of everyday health issues—and with no side effects. This form of therapy has been observed and studied for over 100 years, but chances are you have never heard of it. If you have heard of it, you may not think it works.

For most people, this remedy sounds too good to be true, and that's exactly what pharmaceutical companies would like you to believe. To the medical researchers who have spent years studying and documenting this natural phenomenon, however, the science is clear. The goal of this book is to provide you with a clear understanding of how negative ions work and how you may find tremendous relief through exposure to these tiny therapeutic chemical elements.

The text begins by defining negative ions and explaining how they may work to ease various health disorders. It goes on to look at the history of negative ions, revealing that Nikola Tesla, one the world's most brilliant inventors and researchers, may have been the first person to recognize their effects on people. Readers are then given insight into the specific health conditions that may be relieved or mitigated through exposure to negative-ion therapy and its many benefits, hopefully learning how to use the power of negative ions to overcome their own health issues. This book includes some of the major research on negative ions that has been conducted over the last hundred years, detailing the advantages associated with these fascinating atoms and molecules. Lastly, readers will find a handy reference guide to negative-ion generators, which should provide all the information needed to make an educated decision on which one to use.

Good health may be something you wish for others or for yourself, but wishing doesn't ensure that it will happen. By taking responsibility for your well-being, you may be able to achieve the good health you seek. By learning as much as you can about safe and proven alternative treatments for certain ailments, you may obtain the relief that has thus far been elusive.

I hope this book leads you to a life full of energy, happiness, sound sleep, and rejuvenation, leaving you able to overcome any challenges that may come your way.

1

What Are Negative Ions?

Think back to the most recent time you visited a beach, lake, or even the local park. How did the environment make you feel? Chances are you felt energized, alert, and rejuvenated. That's because in addition to the beautiful scenery and relaxing activities, there were thousands of invisible mood-enhancers all around you called negative ions.

While you may be unaware of it, negative ions are responsible for that sudden rush of feel-good energy you experience when you walk outside for the first time after eight hours in a sterile, air-conditioned office. Depression, mood disorders such as seasonal affective disorder (SAD), and even allergies to spores, pollen, and dust have all been shown to improve with enough exposure to negative ions. The benefits, however, don't stop there. Negative ions may be beneficial in all areas of your personal health and well-being, including sleep, weight loss, concentration, and athletic performance.

This chapter will look at what negative ions are and how their many healthful effects were discovered. As you will learn, the good news is that you don't have to travel all the way to the nearest waterfall to expose yourself to negative ions. In fact, anyone can enjoy the advantages of negative ions, regardless of geographic location. One of the easiest ways to experience the benefits of negative ions would be to drive out to the country, roll down your car window, and breathe in some fresh air. Here's an example that's even closer to home: Take a shower. Don't you feel more awake after a shower? While you may not have realized it, this sense of refreshment is the product of negative ions.

Of course, science has been able to harness the force of these ions in a more controlled manner, as you will find out in Chapter 4. Before we get to that, however, the first thing you should understand is the nature of this amazing electrical wonder.

ION BASICS

In order to understand what ions are and what they do, we must discuss electricity. We can see the power of electricity in our homes as it provides the energy that enables lights to shine, appliances to run, and temperatures to rise and fall according to our needs. The electricity we use at home is carried by wires. The human body is, in a manner of speaking, wired in the same way. Electricity flows through your nervous system, allowing your heart to beat, your skin to feel, and your brain to think. Without this "charge of life," there would be no life—human or otherwise. It is clear that electricity plays an important role in our own abilities to function as well as in the world at large. So, what are the elements that make up electricity? To answer this question, we need to understand a little bit about physics.

The physical world—everything you know—is composed of very tiny chemical elements called atoms. Molecules are formed when two or more atoms are joined together chemically. For example, think of a Lego set. Consider a single Lego piece an atom. When you combine two Lego pieces together, you create a molecule.

At the center of each atom is the nucleus. The nucleus is made up of particles known as protons and neutrons. Protons possess a positive charge, while neutrons do not have any charge. Like moons orbiting a planet, particles called electrons spin around the nucleus. Electrons are negatively charged. When there are an equal number of protons and electrons in an atom, the molecule is said to have a neutral charge. When these particles are unbalanced, the atom or molecule is called an ion and holds either a positive charge or a negative charge. An ion with more protons than electrons is called a positive ion, while an ion with more electrons than protons is called a negative ion. Both positive and negative ions occur naturally but may also be created by man-made devices. Moreover, both types of ion can affect behavior and attitude.

THE POSITIVE IONS AROUND US

Positive ions can be created by hot desert winds, cell phones, radio and television transmitters, cell towers, and direct current power lines. While their effects on humans are controversial, the results of being exposed to too many positive ions do not appear to be good. Arguments can be made that too much exposure to these ions may be detrimental to your health and well-being. Positive ions may even have the potential to increase emotional distress, disrupt brain function, induce problematic metabolic changes, cause fatigue, and interfere with the functions of the immune system. Research seems to indicate that some people may be more prone to the negative effects of positive ions than others.

While the negative effects of positive ions have not been determined conclusively, what we do know is that modern lifestyle has placed all of us in an environment that is permanently creating positive ions. A quick glance around any room in your house will reveal many of these man-made positive-ion generators, such as your cell phone, television, laptop, or air conditioner. Your work environment is likely similar, trapping you in a vicious cycle no matter where you go, and leaving you feeling tired and unmotivated all day long. At the same time, when it comes to office buildings, often a building's insulation is such that it does not allow the inflow of beneficial negative ions to offset all the harmful positive ions being generated inside. Engineers and construction workers go to great lengths to make buildings as insulated as possible, which helps business owners maintain and regulate temperatures inside their offices more easily. The downside to this superior insulation is that it not only prevents negative ions from coming in but also keeps the positive ions from cell phones, microwaves, dust, pollution, and stale air from escaping. The result is poor air quality.

Thankfully, negative ions are much more prevalent in nature than positive ions. They can be found at beaches, by lakes, on mountains, near waterfalls, and after thunderstorms.

NATURE'S NEGATIVE IONS

In nature, the most common molecules include hydrogen, carbon dioxide, oxygen, and water. When a violent natural event, such as a heavy waterfall hitting the surface of a lake, is in the midst of occurring, its sheer force ejects electrons from water molecules and spreads them into the air, where they then search for other molecules on which to cling.

In the waterfall example, the electrons leaving the water molecules tend to attach themselves to oxygen molecules. As mentioned, once an atom or molecule acquires more electrons than it has protons (in this case, extra electrons from the water molecules), it instantly becomes a negative ion. Thus, as the force of the waterfall removes a few electrons from each water molecule, thousands of negatively charged oxygen molecules are created and the air is made rich in negative ions. The sheer number of negative ions in the air you breathe causes you to feel clear and revitalized almost immediately. If you've ever been to a waterfall and taken a deep breath, that surreal alertness and sense of self-awareness is the abundance of negative ions at work. Negative ions can be measured in cubic centimeters, and a typical waterfall setting can have as many as 5,000 negative ions per cubic centimeter. Visit Niagara Falls and you'll experience a whopping 100,000 negative ions per cubic centimeter.

People who suffer the ill effects of airborne allergens receive an added benefit from negative ions. As negative charges attract positive charges, negative ions attract allergens such as dust, mold, and pollen, which are positively charged. The allergens combine with the negative ions, forming clusters that become heavy and fall to the ground to be swept up instead of inhaled.

Sadly, upon returning from any trip during which negative ions were plentiful, you will most probably be welcomed back to an office environment that rewards you with fewer than 50 negative ions per cubic centimeter. And if you leave the air conditioner on or get stuck in traffic during rush hour, that number will plummet to almost zero.

Waterfalls, of course, aren't the only way to experience a healthy dose of negative ions. You can visit the beach and stand near the shore, where the waves crash into the shoreline and are constantly moving. If the weather doesn't warrant a trip to the beach, you can always try the negative ion generator right in your own home: the shower. In the shower, water crashes against the walls and your body, and you are right in the middle of it all. After only ten or fifteen minutes in the shower, you will already feel refreshed and ready to take on the day.

CONCLUSION

While, understandably, the physical action of negative and positive ions cannot be seen by the naked eye, scientists today are able to measure the level of ions made by both natural and artificial means. In spite of the observable changes in human behavior after exposure to negative ions, there has been a great reluctance on the part of the conservative medical community to accept the many benefits provided by these molecules. But why shouldn't we consider as treatment this effective remedy to a host of problems? Negative ions can be self-administered, have no problematic side effects, and cost a great deal less than a daily regimen of drugs to acquire. As you shall see in the next chapter, there is a remarkable history behind the discovery of negative ions and their benefits—one that includes some of the world's greatest minds.

2

A Brief History

It may have been an article written by Nikola Tesla in 1900 that opened the door to understanding the medical benefits of ions, but the power of electricity has always played an important role in the development of human society. It is worth noting that what we take for granted today was a great source of mystery for millennia.

IN THE BEGINNING

Early humans living in caves knew of electricity through the bolts of lightning unleashed from the heavens during thunderstorms. While they may not have understood the science of electricity, they quickly learned to fear and respect this majestic power from above—a power that produced uncommonly loud claps of thunder, split mighty trees in half, started fires, and extinguished the life of any poor soul standing in the wrong place. Over time, this phenomenon would be given a divine quality according to various religious traditions. From the Greeks to the Romans, from the Chinese to the indigenous tribes scattered throughout the world, lightning had a special meaning.

It would take the scientific minds of the Age of Enlightenment of the mid-eighteenth century to give serious thought to understanding the nature of electricity. One of the earliest investigations of lightning was proposed by Benjamin Franklin at the outset of the 1750s. To prove that lightning was, indeed, electricity, Franklin suggested flying a kite with a key attached to it in the middle of a thunderstorm. Although we do not know that Franklin actually performed this famous experiment, as the story goes, he mounted a piece of wire to the kite as a lightning rod, and then attached a key to the bottom of the kite string, which was connected to a Leyden jar. This jar would be used to "collect" the electricity from the lightning. During a storm, he noticed the wet string of the kite being charged with static electricity and decided to touch the key, receiving a mild shock. This shock, along with witnessing the electrified string and subsequently charged Leyden jar, was proof that lightning was, in fact, a form of electricity. Moreover, Franklin was the first to theorize the cause of a bolt of lightning as the exchange of a negative force and a positive force. Based on these notions, Franklin would invent the lightning rod, which would be used to protect structures from catching fire as a result of lightning strikes.

In Europe, additional theories were soon being devised and experiments conducted in an effort to better understand this force of nature. In the 1770s, Father Giuseppe Toaldo, a famous Italian physicist and professor, influenced by Benjamin Franklin's new invention, decided to measure electricity's impact on plant growth. He claimed that plants growing next to a lightning rod's conductor wire grew almost ten times taller than identical plants only a few feet away. In 1775, Father Giovanni Battista Beccaria of the University of Turin set out to determine if electricity had an observable effect on plant life as well. In his *Treatise upon Artificial Electricity,* he wrote, "With regard to atmospheric electricity it appears manifest, that nature makes and extensive use of it for promoting vegetation." These were the first steps towards recognition of electricity's influence on the natural world and all living things.

At about the same time, French physicist Jean-Antoine Nollet, the first to be named professor of physics at the University of Paris, planted several dozen mustard seeds in two separate containers and electrified one of the containers using an electrostatic generator. At the end of one week, every seed in the electrified container had sprouted and grown a few millimeters, while the other container showed little progress. While these experiments showed that the use of static electricity improved the growth of plants, the underlying physics of electricity would not be explored until the mid-1800s.

In 1830s England, Michael Faraday documented the movements of ions as he studied electrical charges in gas-filled tubes, which were essentially early versions of cathode tubes. And while scientists throughout Europe were debating the nature of these particles, it was Julius Elster and Hans Friedrich Geitel, two lifelong friends and physics teachers working together at the Great School of Wolfenbüttel in Germany, who stated that electrostatic fields were made up of the electrically charged particles known as ions, which could be found in the air all around us. Their discovery would be one of the first major steps towards realizing just how electrically charged our environment really is.

TESLA OPENS THE DOOR

It would take the vision of an engineering genius to refine the electrical system we use today as well as to recognize the true power of negative ions. Nikola Tesla was born in Serbia in 1856. After studying physics and engineering at the Austrian Polytechnic Institute in Graz and the University of Prague in the 1870s, he immigrated to the United States in 1884. First working at Thomas Edison's laboratory in 1884, Tesla soon left Edison's employ, feeling mistreated by his American employer, who was much more focused on business success and finances than on real technical advancements in electrical engineering.

With the financial backing of other supporters, Tesla would develop technologies to generate and transmit alternating-current (AC) electricity, experiment with x-rays and radio communication, and work with General Electric to create the

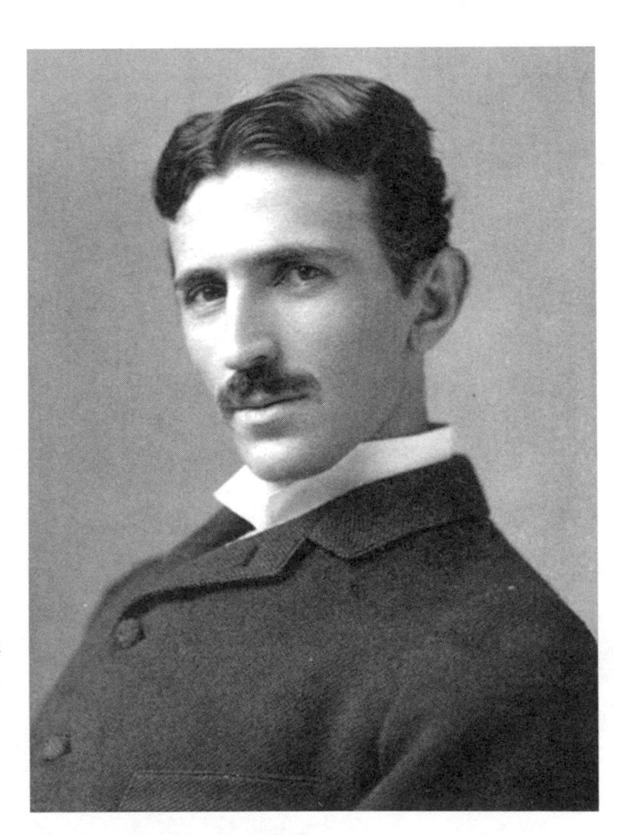

Nikola Tesla
Born in Serbia in 1856, Nikola Tesla studied physics and engineering at the Austrian Polytechnic Institute in Graz and the University of Prague in the 1870s, and immigrated to the United States in 1884. This photo shows Tesla at thirty-four years old, one year before he would invent the Tesla coil.

first modern power station at Niagara Falls. While his interests were many and varied, he devoted a great deal of research to the study of the electrical properties involved in x-rays, wireless communication, ionization, electromagnetic flux, and Earth's field of gravity.

Tesla's most widely known invention may be the high-voltage transformer known as the "Tesla coil," which he created in 1891, after conducting dangerous experiments that involved hundreds of thousands of volts of electricity. According to Margaret Cheney's *Tesla: Man Out of Time,* these experiments led Tesla to announce "the therapeutic deep-heating value of high-frequency currents on the human body," which would initiate the creation of "an enormous field of medical technology, with many early imitators both in America and Europe." While this field of technology was mainly focused on the possible medical uses of "heat production resulting from the bombardment of tissue with high-frequency alternating currents," which today include x-ray, microwave, and radio wave applications, Tesla was also interested in the health benefits of what he called "cold fire." This "cold fire" was essentially the brush discharge from a low-power device, which Tesla felt both refreshed the mind and cleansed the skin. In fact, he may have been simply describing the effects of negative ions.

Perhaps Tesla's most notable depiction of the power of negative ions came as a result of his disappointment at being bested by German scientist Carl von Linde. After Linde reported his breakthrough in the process of liquefying oxygen—a process on which Tesla himself had been working—Tesla became depressed. As described by author Margaret Cheney, the inventor relied on his "electric treatment" to overcome his sadness, stating:

> I was so blue and discouraged in those days . . . that I don't believe I could have borne up but for the regular electric treatment which I administered to myself. You see, electricity puts into the tired body just what it most needs—life force, nerve force. It's a great doctor, I can tell you, perhaps the greatest of all doctors.

Although Tesla was not at all interested in turning his small Tesla coil into a business in the field of medical equipment, he allowed a third party to produce and sell these devices to the doctors and professors who had been phoning in from all over the country with inquiries. Sales of his medical coil soon brought him some money, which he used to finance new inventions.

In its June 1900 issue, *The Century* boasted a "remarkable article by Nikola Tesla," "The Problem of Increasing Human Energy." [See page 18.] In this piece, Tesla discussed his machine, the Tesla coil, and the way in which it allowed electrical current to flow through the air. Technology at that time had been using wire to conduct electricity, as technology still does today, but Tesla had been able to use air. In connection with this phenomenon, Tesla also described a remarkable feat. He had allowed the electricity being carried through the air to pass through his body with absolutely no harmful effects. He had "demonstrated that powerful electrical discharges of several hundred thousand volts, which at that time were considered absolutely deadly, could be passed through the body without inconvenience or hurtful consequences."

While this description would surely have been enough to thrill readers, Tesla mentioned another significant observation in his article. To quote the inventor, "These oscillations produced other specific physiological effects, which, upon my

THE JUNE
CENTURY
CONTAINS A
REMARKABLE
ARTICLE BY
NIKOLA
TESLA
THE ELECTRICAL
INVENTOR
FROM THE JUNE CENTURY
ON
INCREASING
HUMAN ENERGY
WITH
ANNOUNCEMENT OF NEW DISCOVERIES

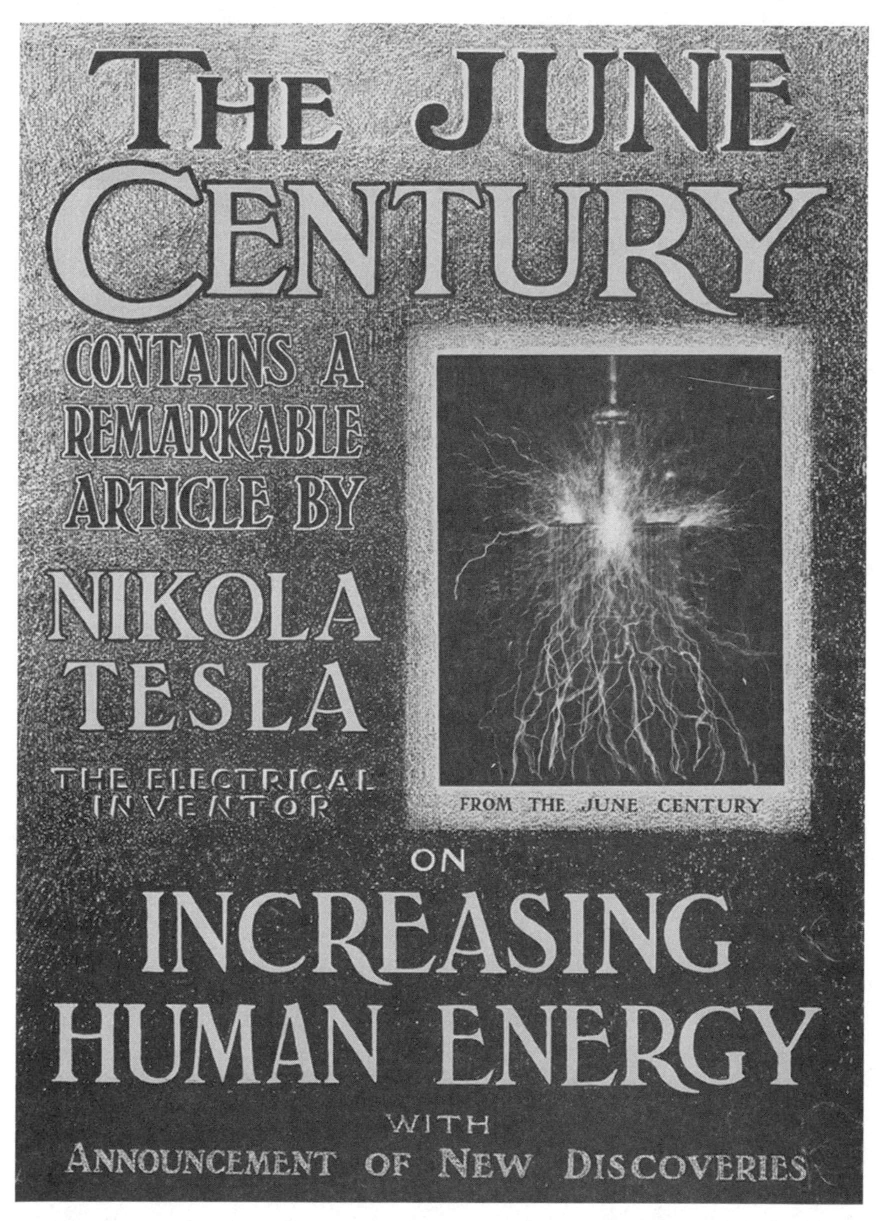

Beginning as a small Christian publication, *The Century* magazine became the largest periodical in the country by the late nineteenth century, focusing on a wider and more generally educated audience. The June 1900 issue included a "remarkable article by Nikola Tesla," "The Problem of Increasing Human Energy," which discussed the Tesla coil, a machine that allowed electrical current to flow through the air.

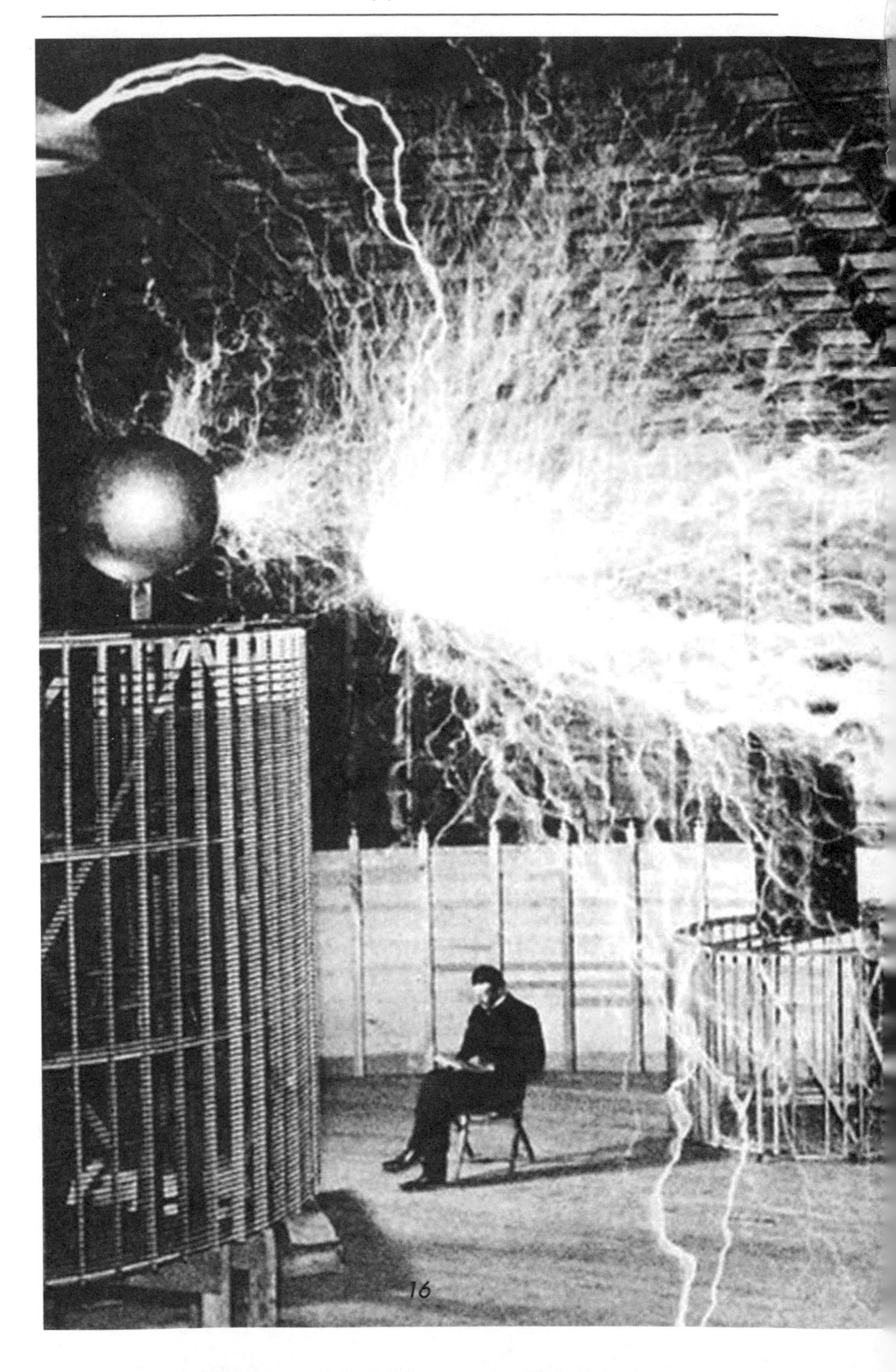

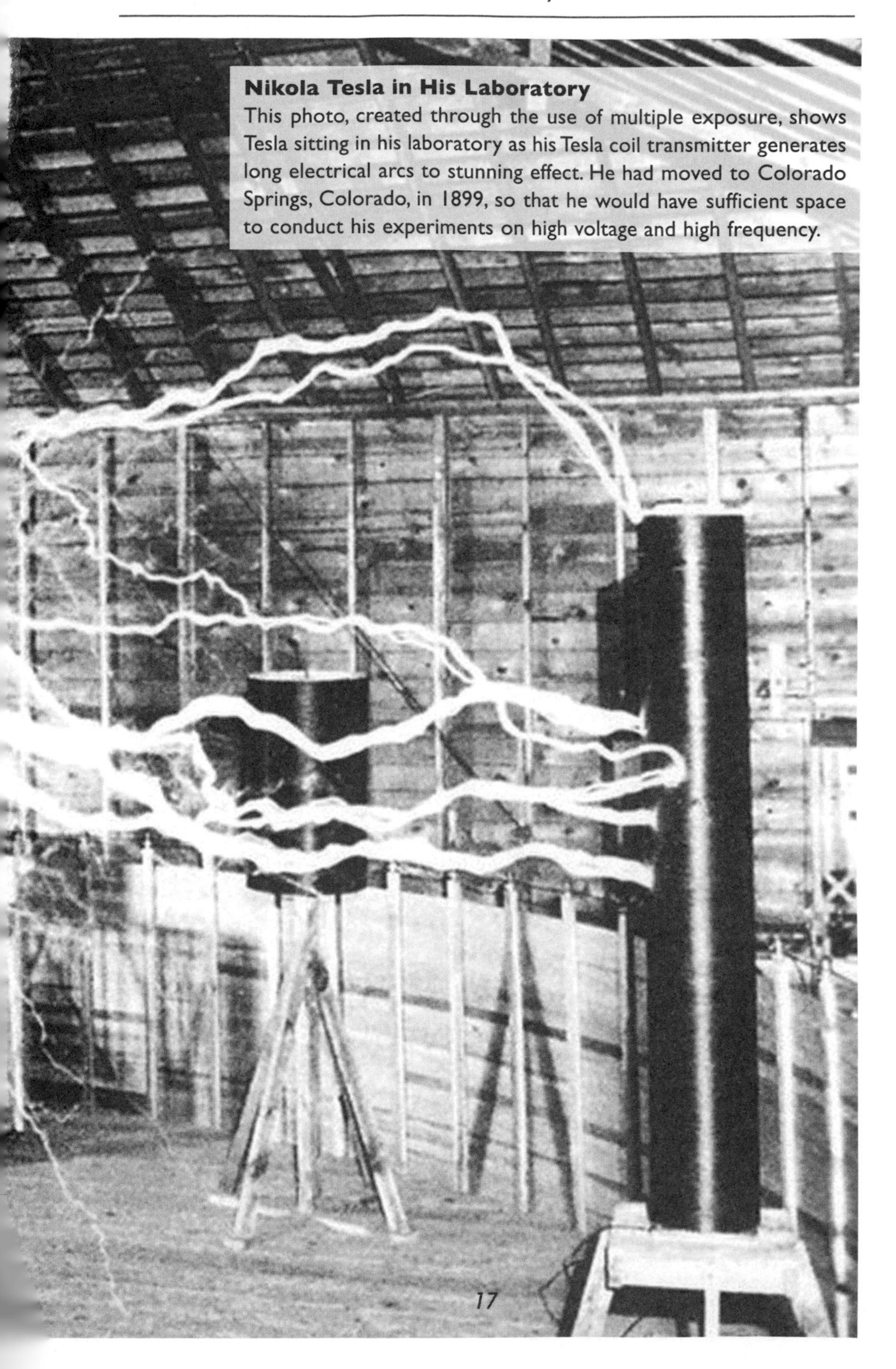

Nikola Tesla in His Laboratory
This photo, created through the use of multiple exposure, shows Tesla sitting in his laboratory as his Tesla coil transmitter generates long electrical arcs to stunning effect. He had moved to Colorado Springs, Colorado, in 1899, so that he would have sufficient space to conduct his experiments on high voltage and high frequency.

From "The Problem of Increasing Human Energy" by Nikola Tesla

The Century, June 1900 issue

"The discovery of the conducting properties of the air, though unexpected, was only a natural result of experiments in a special field which I had carried on for some years before. It was, I believe, during 1889 that certain possibilities offered by extremely rapid electrical oscillations determined me to design a number of special machines adapted for their investigation. Owing to the peculiar requirements, the construction of these machines was very difficult, and consumed much time and effort; but my work on them was generously rewarded, for I reached by their means several novel and important results. One of the earliest observations I made with these new machines was that electrical oscillations of an extremely high rate act in an extraordinary manner upon the human organism. Thus, for instance, I demonstrated that powerful electrical discharges of several hundred thousand volts, which at that time were considered absolutely deadly, could be passed through the body without inconvenience or hurtful consequences. **These oscillations produced other specific physiological effects, which, upon my announcement, were eagerly taken up by skilled physicians and further investigated. This new field has proved itself fruitful beyond expectation, and in the few years which have passed since, it has been developed to such an extent that it now forms a legitimate and important department of medical science.** Many results, thought impossible at that time, are now readily obtainable with these oscillations, and many experiments undreamed of then can now be readily performed by their means. I still remember with pleasure how, nine years ago, I passed the discharge of a powerful induction-coil through my body to demonstrate before a scientific society the comparative harmlessness of very rapidly vibrating electric currents, and I can still recall the astonishment of my audience. I would now undertake, with much less apprehension that I had in that experiment, to transmit through my body with such currents the entire electrical energy of the dynamos now working at Niagara—forty or fifty thousand horse-power. I have produced electrical oscillations which were of such intensity that when circulating through my arms and chest they have melted wires which joined my hands, and still I felt no inconvenience. I have energized with such oscillations a loop of heavy copper wire so powerfully that masses of metal, and even objects of an electrical resistance specifically greater than that of human tissue brought close to or placed within the loop, were heated to a high temperature and melted, often with the violence of an explosion, and yet into this very space in which this terribly-destructive turmoil was going on I have repeatedly thrust my head without feeling anything or experiencing injurious after-effects."

announcement, were eagerly taken up by skilled physicians and further investigated. This new field has proved itself fruitful beyond expectation, and in the few years which have passed since, it has been developed to such an extent that it now forms a legitimate and important department of medical science." Using electrical currents emanating from his Tesla coil, it seems Tesla had been able to create positive ions and negative ions—something that had not been done before, or, at least, had not been recognized by the scientific community at the time. Most likely, Tesla was referring to the physiological effects brought about by exposure to the negative ions generated during his experiment—the very same ions that hold the potential to heal the body and change an individual's attitude. Unfortunately, Tesla never built upon the potential of these findings, though he had been fascinated with them at the time. Instead, he chose other paths to follow—ones that met his ever-changing interests.

Despite giving very little attention to his coil's medical applications, "[i]n his old age Tesla was gratified to hear his invention of electrical oscillation devices for medical therapy receive high accolades." The truth is that the therapeutic implications of Tesla's work are still being explored in the medical field. "As is typical of so many of Tesla's inventions, scholars still do not know the whole range of their possible applications."

THE WORK OF DR. HANSELL

It was not until the early 1930s that the first specific investigation into the biological effects of ionized air began, thanks to an American research engineer named Dr. Clarence Hansell. An inventor of extraordinary merit, Dr. Hansell founded and directed the Rocky Point Research Section of the RCA Radio Transmission Laboratory in 1925, and by the time of his death in 1967, had been granted over 300 US patents, second only to Thomas Edison.

As Dr. Hansell worked in his laboratory in 1932, he noticed something peculiar in the behavior of one of his laboratory assistant engineers. When his assistant worked next to the electrostatic generator, he seemed to experience mood swings whenever the generator changed its polarity and thus the type of ions it released into the air. If the generator produced negative ions, the assistant felt a sense of euphoria and was more energetic. When the machine made positive ions, however, the assistant would experience a drop in mood and would easily become aggressive and be more prone to headaches. Hansell

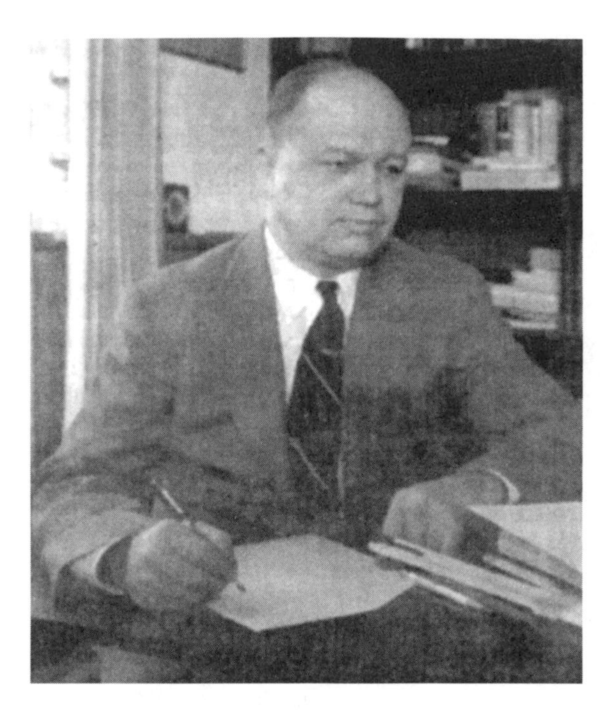

Dr. Clarence Hansell
Dr. Clarence Hansell founded and directed the Rocky Point Research Section of the RCA Radio Transmission Laboratory in 1925, and by the time of his death in 1967, had been granted over 300 US patents, second only to Thomas Edison. His laboratory observations in 1932 led to his pioneering research on negative ions and their therapeutic effects.

reasoned that this behavior change was more than likely due to one thing—the type of ions being generated by the lab's large generator. He clearly recognized that the ionized air had produced a powerful biological effect on his assistant. But there was more.

As he studied his engineer's behavior, Dr. Hansell observed something else that was just as intriguing. The lab he worked in was always full of dust, owing to all the activities that were going on. For those who suffered from allergies, the particles floating in the air only made their conditions worse. As soon as the ion generator began producing negative ions, however, something amazing happened. Those allergy sufferers who were closest to the generator experienced the complete disappearance of their symptoms. The more Dr. Hansell observed this phenomenon, the more he came to realize that it was the negative ions that could not only alter mood but also alleviate allergies by eliminating the offending specks from the air.

Working with his machinist, Al Streib, Dr. Hansell created a small mobile device that could produce negative ions. He and Streib tested their machine on family members and friends, and could quickly see how effective it was at getting rid of airborne allergens and boosting mood. Over the next few years, Dr. Hansell approached the executives at RCA, asking them to consider producing a similar tool, but RCA saw no value in its commercial production.

In 1945, Dr. Hansell served as a scientific investigator with the Technical Industrial Intelligence Committee in Germany for the US Government. His interest in ions had not waned. While there, he continued to investigate and report on information concerning air ionization. He theorized that by putting a negative-ion device in submarines, he could reduce the amount of allergies in the air of the vessel and improve the moods of the sailors.

This ionization theory led to an association with Mr. W. Wesley Hicks, President of Wesix Electric Heater Company. Mr. Hicks soon became one of the most active promoters and the most effective supporter of air ionization research in the United States. Their association continued until the death of Mr. Hicks on December 8, 1960. It was Mr. Hicks' involvement in the commercial application of negative-ion equipment that opened up the field for the introduction of artificially ionized air produced by air conditioners.

As Hicks was developing negative-ion equipment, Hansell continued to research and write about the therapeutic potential of negative ions until his death. Unfortunately for both Hicks and Hansell, the work on negative ions in the US came under attack as quackery by the medical establishment throughout the post-war era, in spite of the existence of evidence to the contrary. Whatever negative ion research done or equipment created in the United States, it was quickly labeled fraudulent by the mainstream scientific community.

Along with a handful of European nations, it was predominantly the Soviet Union that resumed government-sanctioned studies on electricity and ionization soon after the war. It was Russian pride and emphasis on its athletes that led their researchers to continue the work on negative ions. Their immediate goal was to see how effective it could be in improving their athletes' performance abilities.

CONCLUSION

As historical record proves, while scientists of the eighteenth century sensed the connection between electricity and its influence on life—specifically plant life—it was scientists of the early twentieth century who came to understand the physical nature of negative ions. Beyond the real breakthroughs that both Tesla and Hansell had made in connection with ions and human behavior, however, the potential of ionized air was brushed under the carpet in the United States. While emphasis in this country focused on finding magic potions in the form of pharmaceuticals to cure a wide range of illnesses, other scientists from around the world looked towards the fascinating subject of ions for better, safer, and more concrete answers.

3

Health Benefits of Negative-Ion Exposure

One of the greatest economic issues facing our nation today is the growing cost of healthcare. While the number of patients being treated for degenerative illnesses continues to increase, their medical care costs have skyrocketed—and that's not including the rising cost of health insurance coverage. If a safe, effective, and money-saving complementary treatment could be used to combat the same disorders that are costing our nation billions of dollars annually, wouldn't it be a prudent decision to use it?

By the early 1950s, hundreds of compelling studies on the positive effects of negative ions were being carried out by scientists and medical researchers throughout the world. Each study had a similar theme: Excessive positive ionization can cause many unwanted side effects, while negative ions may provide energy, a sense of well-being, and numerous other health benefits.

This chapter lists a number of common health issues and how they may be alleviated through the use of negative-ion exposure. At the outset of negative-ion treatment, some people may feel relief immediately. For others, it may come in gradual stages. For still others, the changes they're looking for may not come at all. This treatment should not be considered a magical cure-all. You are the best judge when it comes to determining how well negative ions work for you. Unlike the potential problems associated with drug treatments, however, you can rest assured there will be no troublesome side effects from negative-ion therapy.

ALLERGIES AND ASTHMA

Do you suffer from allergies or asthma? According to the Asthma and Allergy Foundation of America (AAFA), a non-profit organization founded in the early 1950s, approximately one in five Americans suffer from allergy or asthma symptoms. Even with modern advances in medicine and technology, the number of asthma cases has continued to rise since 1980, regardless of age, race, or sex. Worse still, a little over half of the population of the United States tests positive to at least one or more allergen. Although the reason for this increase remains unclear, some factors likely responsible include air pollution, obesity, poor diet, and decreased physical activity.

There are two more factors that may be playing a role in the rising cases of allergies and asthma, but they are more difficult to measure: A decrease in indoor air ventilation from air-tight construction and a much higher count of positive ions due to man-made electronics and machinery. In fact, according to the Environmental Protection Agency (EPA), "indoor levels of pollutants may be 2 to 5 times—and occasionally more than 100 times—higher than outdoor pollutant levels." The EPA also states that indoor air pollutants are actually one of the top five environmental risks to public health, and that "the average American spends approximately 90 percent of their time indoors."

Look through a ray of light shining through your window to get a brief glimpse of what you are breathing in. Fresh country air has about 6,000 particles floating in every milliliter, while the air we breathe in and around a typical city can have several million particles per milliliter. With so much time spent indoors, you can see how easily health complications, however subtle, may occur.

It is well known that air pollution can be damaging to the lungs. Not many people realize, however, that high levels of pollution in the air may also affect the heart. The Environmental Protection Agency (EPA) officially considers it a threat to cardiovascular health, in fact. In early 2002, a large and robust study involving 500,000 individuals was published in the *Journal of the American Medical Association.* The study revealed that during sudden increases in air pollution levels, incidents of death related to health conditions such as pneumonia, asthma, and emphysema rose. According to the EPA, more than 5 percent of heart disease deaths are possibly connected to air pollution exposure.

One study, which was published in the April 2013 issue of *PLOS Medicine,* had more than 5,000 men and women participate in ultrasound examinations that measured one of two arteries responsible for carrying oxygenated blood to the head and neck area. Each subject was followed for two and a half years, with researchers measuring the thickness of each subject's artery as well as air pollution data on the concentration of floating particulate matter. The scientists found that as the levels of air pollution got higher, the artery became thicker, regardless of the subject's race, gender, education level, or smoking history.

Negatively charged ions can help remove allergens and pollutants from the air. That's because many of these floating particles have either a neutral or a positive charge. Because opposites attract, negative ions stick to particles of dust, mold, pet dander, pollen, and other allergens. These clusters of negative ions and air pollutants clump together until they become heavy enough that gravity causes them to fall to the ground, where they may be vacuumed up. Negative-ion generators are even effective against viruses and bacteria in the air. Among the many studies showing the ability of negative ions to reduce airborne contaminants is a 2001 paper by the US Department of Agriculture (USDA), which stated that "high levels of negative air ions can have a significant impact on the airborne microbial load . . . [and] also causes significant reduction in airborne dust. . . . Other potential applications include any enclosed space such as food processing areas, medical institutions, the workplace, and the home, where reduction of airborne and surface pathogens is desired." A 2002 study done by the USDA found that negative-ion technology reduced airborne bacteria and dust within a poultry hatching cabinet. Negative ions lowered bacteria levels by 85 to 93 percent, while dust levels experienced a reduction of 93 percent.

In 1966, a study published in *Pediatrics* reported the results of a series of tests on thirty-eight infants between the ages of two and twelve months old. Each infant had almost the same degree of breathing problems. The children were divided into two groups of nineteen. One group was used as a control group and placed in a room where ion generators would not be utilized, while the other group was placed in a ward where negative-ion generators would be turned on. The control group would be treated with drugs and antibiotics, the other group would not. The results were astonishing. The group that

Air Pollution and Child Development

According to the EPA, adults may develop health complications from exposure to air pollution, ranging from mild symptoms such as skin rash, throat irritation, and headache to more serious symptoms, including nervous system damage, chronic bronchitis, and cancer. Unfortunately, research studies have shown that children are much more susceptible to air pollution than adults. There are several reasons why children respond differently to air pollution as compared to adults. One important difference is that children breathe more air at any given level of exertion. During competitive sports, for example, a child can breathe between 20 and 50 percent more air than an adult. This results in more air pollutants being inhaled, causing the child's body to absorb higher concentrations of pollution.

Another difference is that children typically don't show the same symptoms associated with air pollution as adults, and many times they don't show any signs at all, making the issue tough to recognize. It's currently not known if the reason for this reality is that children don't acknowledge their symptoms or that they just ignore them because they are too preoccupied with other matters.

Children do not have fully developed lungs, which could be problematic if they are exposed to high levels of air pollution. Cells that are important in the development of strong lungs can be severely damaged if exposed to air pollution, and the lungs may not be able to achieve full growth or function due to air pollution, leaving the child with permanently weak lungs.

was exposed to negative ions saw its symptoms eliminated much quicker than the symptoms of the infants who were not exposed to negative ions. This result was achieved without any other treatment. Additionally, no negative side effects were experienced by the group of infants that did not receive drugs or antibiotics. In contrast, a 1984 study published in *Thorax* evaluated the effect of positive ions on twelve asthmatic children challenged by exercise. Positively ionized air was shown to significantly aggravate exercise-induced asthma, worsening bronchial response to exercise in the children.

Many studies seem to suggest that by decreasing positive ions in the air and increasing negative ions, levels of airborne particulate matter can be reduced and breathing problems alleviated. According to a report published in 1977, negative ions appear capable of counteracting the allergenic effects positive ions can have on respiratory tissues. This finding supports Krueger and Smith's research done in 1958, which stated that negative-ion exposure increased ciliary activity in the trachea. Cilia are tiny filaments that line the human bronchial tubes and trachea (also known as the windpipe). They move in a back-and-forth motion designed to clear dust, pollen, and other airborne contaminants from the body's air passages. As you might have expected, according to the same report, positive ions decreased ciliary activity.

ADHD

According to a study by Craig Garfield at Northwestern University, more American children are being diagnosed with ADHD (Attention Deficit Hyperactivity Disorder) than ever before, placing the current number at approximately 10.4 million children in 2010. That's up 66 percent from 2000, just ten years earlier. ADHD is a disorder that changes a person's ability to focus, and typical symptoms associated with ADHD include disruptive behavior, inattentiveness, distractibility, anxiety, reduced cognitive thinking, daydreaming, and constant procrastination. Though there is no single test that detects ADHD, diagnosis is a long process that involves several steps, and patients need to display at least six or more symptoms over a six-month period.

Just as they can help everyday concentration, negative ions may have a similarly positive effect on children with ADHD. By providing more oxygen to the brain and encouraging proper serotonin levels, negative ions may help a child with ADHD feel more alert and able to concentrate. A study published by the *Journal of Abnormal Child Psychology* in 1984 reported the effect of negative-ion therapy on children with learning disabilities. According to the research, the children exposed to an environment rich in negative ions displayed improved incidental memory and selective attention. In 1990, the same researchers published a study in the *International Journal of Biometeorology,* which also showed the possible remedial applications of negative ions in regard to some learning-challenged youngsters.

A learning experiment published by the *International Journal of Biometeorology* in 1969 tested the effects of negative ions on a group of rats tasked to navigate a maze. Results showed that those rats exposed to fifteen minutes of increased levels of negative ions each day over a period of two weeks displayed fewer errors and improved time scores, suggesting a strong link between this therapy and the ability to learn.

HEALING AND THE IMMUNE SYSTEM

Negative ions may also boost the immune system and help the body heal itself. In 1959, a researcher named Dr. Igho H. Kornblueh treated 138 burn victims at the Northeastern General Hospital with negatively charged air. What he found was that almost 60 percent of the burn victims experienced a significant reduction in pain and discomfort, while at the same time healed faster and more thoroughly. On the other hand, only 22 percent of a control group that underwent traditional burn treatments had similar results. Along with his colleagues Gualtierotti and Sirtori, Kornblueh published another report on the healing power of negative ions in 1968, in which 138 burn victims noted reduced pain levels and quick scar tissue formation after receiving negative-ion therapy. The hastening of the healing process may have been due to the ability of negative ions to prevent microorganism infection.

In defense of this idea, a 1986 study published in *General Physiology and Biophysics* showed accelerated wound healing in rats whose skin had been deprived of epidermis and then exposed to negative ions for three hours. Conversely, positive-ion exposure slowed healing. According to the same scientists behind this research, soft tissue deprived of oxygen promotes the growth of harmful microorganisms such *Clostridium perfringens* and *Staphylococcus aureus,* both of which are killed by negative ions pulsed on the injured tissue. In fact, in 1979, the *Journal of Hygiene* had already declared this particular benefit of negative-ion exposure, publishing a study that showed reductions in bacterial levels in hospital burn units after two weeks of filling these environments with high levels of negative ions. These reductions resulted in quicker and better healing in patients.

In 2002, an article in *Critical Care Medicine* detailed the effects of negative-ion exposure on postoperative recovery. It stated that patients who had received negative-ion therapy after surgery displayed faster rates of recovery than those who had not. In addition to aiding recovery, negative ions seem to prevent certain types of injury as well, as evidenced by a 1975 study in which negative ions helped irradiated animals avoid radiation injuries.

Mucosal surfaces inside the body, such as the gastrointestinal tract and the respiratory tract, produce approximately 15 percent of the body's Immunoglobulin A, or IgA, which is the principal antibody in their secretions. Antibodies, of course, are proteins used by the immune system to fight off unwanted bacteria and viruses in the body. According to a 2004 study published in the *International Journal of Occupational Medicine and Environmental Health,* negative ions can elevate levels of salivary immunoglobulin A, which illustrates the mechanism behind their ability to promote healing and immunity.

In relation to this function, researchers Bordas and Deleanu's 1989 study proved the favorable influence negative ions can have on gastric ulcers. After inducing gastric ulcers in rat test subjects by means of the causative bacteria *Helicobacter pylori,* Bordas and Deleanu treated certain groups with negative ions. They found that those groups treated with negative ions experienced accelerated healing of ulcers, diminished acid secretion and gastric bleeding, and reductions in the sizes of ulcers. The same authors published a follow-up study in 1991, which found that negative-ion therapy significantly decreased the number of ulcers in test animals, promoting durable healing and less gastric pain.

In 2008, Japanese researchers found that negatively charged air could activate the immune system, smooth blood flow, and stabilize the autonomic nervous system. As a result, these scientists also called for analysis of the long-term effects of artificially created negative ions, likely in the hope of recommending the use of negative-ion generators to improve the indoor atmosphere of places high in positive ions, such as office buildings, in the future. An office building with a negative-ion generator may see a reduction in absenteeism due to illness and an improvement in productivity.

The True Benefits of Breathing Fresh Air

Have you ever wondered what the difference is between normal, everyday air and "fresh" air? Why do you travel to local parks or beaches just to breathe in fresh air? That is exactly the question Dr. Bernell E. Baldwin set out to answer in an article published by *The Journal of Health and Healing* called "Why Is Fresh Air Fresh?" A consultant and instructor in applied physiology at a lifestyle center and hospital for over thirty years, Dr. Baldwin wrote the piece to explain that fresh air is indeed much different than the recirculated air you breathe in every day at home or in the office. Fresh air is full of negative ions, which can revitalize you and improve your overall well-being.

When you work with others in a confined area such as an office building, the same air gets inhaled and exhaled again and again. Over the course of a normal eight-hour work day, you will have breathed in the same recirculated air as everyone else in the office numerous times. Add to this fact the unfortunate reality that most buildings don't leave all the windows open to air out every night, and you could actually be breathing in much of the same polluted air day in and day out! This recirculated air is stale and devoid of any actual freshness, and the pollutants floating around in it are recycled throughout your body each and every day.

Dr. Baldwin's article aligns with the Environmental Protection Agency's warning that indoor air is actually two to five times more polluted than outdoor air. (See page 26.) If the air indoors could be altered to be more like the fresh air we inhale in natural settings, the quality of our work lives would increase dramatically. A case of the Mondays would quickly be erased as your mood and spirit lift and your whole body experiences a decrease in anxiety and an increase in relaxation.

PAIN

Neurotransmitters are chemicals that relay signals between cells in the body, facilitating the communication of information throughout the brain and body. Serotonin, or 5-hydroxytryptamine (5-HT), is a neurotransmitter found mainly in the gastrointestinal tract, blood platelets, and central nervous system. Most of the body's serotonin is used to help keep the digestive system running properly, while the remainder takes part in regulating a wide variety of feelings, overall mood, appetite, and sleep.

Unfortunately, as a chemical designed to transmit signals across neurons, serotonin in the blood seems also to play a large role in the sensation of physical pain. (If you've ever wondered why the sting of a certain spider, hornet, scorpion, or stingray hurts so much, serotonin is a large part of the answer. Some species of these creatures have stingers that inject huge doses of serotonin into the bloodstreams of their unwitting victims.) While the exact mechanisms behind the perception and transmission of pain with the body are still not fully understood, there is scientific data that suggests serotonin in the blood increases pain sensation.

Negative ions help lower serotonin levels in the blood. It seems they do so by speeding up oxidation of this neurotransmitter in the blood, converting it into a biologically inactive form. This may be one of the reasons why so many studies have found a pain-relieving quality to negative-ion therapy. Research on burn victims has shown that exposure to negative ions helps reduce pain levels while also working against infection. Some researchers have even seen benefits associated with cancer patients, who are often in pain. According to one report, cancer patients exposed to ion therapy required less analgesia and experienced accelerated healing of wounds.

For a number of decades, doctors have suggested multiple theories about serotonin's exact role in migraine headaches. Many migraine sufferers will acknowledge disturbances in their stress levels, appetites, moods, and sleep habits as associated characteristics of these painful headaches. Many studies have shown that serotonin-containing neurons in the brainstem are involved in regulating many of these common aspects of human behavior, so it is no wonder that doctors have been considering serotonin's part in migraines and how they might modulate this neurotransmitter to treat this problem.

The specific role of serotonin remains a matter of controversy. For years, scientists have linked migraines to either expanding or constricting blood vessels on the brain's surface. The choice of treatment has also been a source of debate. Drugs that stimulate certain serotonin receptors seem to be effective in the treatment of acute attacks in progress, while drugs that block other serotonin receptors seem effective preventative treatments for migraine. One migraine pain theory, however, states that migraine pain is a result of overactive groups of brain cells that trigger high levels of chemicals such as serotonin. These elevated levels of serotonin constrict blood vessels throughout the body, causing migraine symptoms.

This theory accords with the idea that negative ions, which lower serotonin levels in the blood, may be used to prevent both migraines and headaches in general. According to a 1981 study in the *Journal of Environmental Psychology,* the introduction of a negative-ion generator into an office environment that had been found to be deficient in these ions reduced the complaint rate for headache by 50 percent and significantly decreased the number of reports of nausea and dizziness. In this same office, night-shift working was also associated with headaches and ill-health. Moreover, negative ions seemed to reduce these issues even more effectively at night than during the day. A similar report out of Surrey University described the effect of a negative-ion generator on workers in an office's computer and data collection section. After exposure to an atmosphere rich in negative ions, the workers claimed a reduction in the number of headaches of 78 percent. In addition, the group's job performance improved by 28 percent. Any business owner would be thrilled by these numbers.

MOOD

Similar to the story of Dr. Hansell's laboratory assistant who suffered from mood swings and aggression due to excessive positive ion exposure, other studies continue today regarding ions and the effect they may have on mood and mental health. According to the National Institute of Mental Health, almost 10 percent of the entire population of the United States (about 32 million adults) suffers from at least one type of mood disorder. Although experts are not completely sure of what causes mood disorders such as depression, it is believed that both nature and nurture play roles. While depression often runs in families, its cause may not always be genetic. Stressful or traumatic life events are known to trigger depression. In addition, restlessness, trouble sleeping, and subtle pain—all of which may be caused by a mixture of pollution and positive ions—can also lead to depression.

Depression comes in many different forms. In order to be diagnosed with major depression, you must suffer from five or more depression symptoms for at least two weeks. Major depression typically continues for six months or more if left untreated. Minor depression is similar to major depression but requires only two to four symptoms for a diagnosis.

Dysthymia is a less common form of depression that tends to be more subtle and produces milder symptoms than major or minor depression. This form of depression, however, can easily go untreated for years because its signs are harder to see. Seasonal affective disorder (SAD) is a type of depression that, as its name implies, is usually seasonal. Patients typically begin showing signs of depression in the fall and continue to do so until spring or early summer.

It can be difficult to distinguish SAD symptoms from other types of depression, but generally people affected by SAD have a tendency to feel moody, irate, anxious, and grumpy, and lose interest in things they would have normally enjoyed. Additionally, SAD can cause you to eat more, crave bad foods loaded with calories and carbohydrates, and gain weight. Even though medical experts aren't exactly sure what causes seasonal affective disorder, it is strongly believed that a lack of sunlight may be a factor. After all, lose enough sunlight and you could upset your circadian rhythm, which is the biological clock that tells your body to get sleepy when it's dark out and wake up when it's light. A lack of sunlight could also wreak havoc on the mood-affecting neurotransmitter serotonin. If negative ions can have a positive effect on the regulation of serotonin, perhaps they could counteract the symptoms felt by people affected by SAD.

Interestingly, summer air has a much higher concentration of negative ions compared to winter air, which tends to contain more positive ions. When negative ion generators create enough negative ions to mimic the summer air, those affected by SAD may feel significant improvements in their moods and circadian rhythms. Several studies on this subject have been led by Columbia University professor Dr. Michael Terman. Dr. Terman, who specializes in sleep and depression, holds a doctorate in physiological psychology from Brown University and leads the Center for Light Treatment and Biological Rhythms at Columbia Presbyterian Medical Center as well as the Clinical Chronobiology Program at the New York State Psychiatric Institute. When asked about negative-ion therapy, Dr. Terman responded by saying that negative ion exposure "evokes beneficial mood effects. Although the ions emitted from the machines are not perceptible to your senses, studies have indicated clear improvement in patients with winter depression."

For almost a decade, Dr. Terman and his wife and research assistant Jiuan Su, PhD, have been analyzing the effects of negative ionization and comparing them to more traditional forms of SAD therapy such as bright light and simulated sun exposure. In a 2006 study, ninety-nine adults stricken with seasonal affective disorder were separated into five groups. Each group was assigned a different type of treatment and then treated daily for three weeks. Some of these treatments included exposure to bright light for a half an hour after waking, a steady pulse of light-mimicking dawn for thirteen minutes before waking up, and a simulated sunrise around normal wake-up time. The last two groups were exposed to negative ion generators. One received negative ions at a low-flow rate (low enough not to disturb air circulation) for an hour and a half before waking up, while the other received negative ions for the same length of time, but at a high-flow rate, which Dr. Terman called an "industrial strength" flow rate.

Results from the study, which were published by the *American Journal of Psychiatry*, concluded that negative-ion generators with high-flow rates provide positive outcomes comparable to traditional bright light therapy and antidepressants, but that negative-ion generators with low-flow rates did not have any effect on the subjects. These results echoed outcomes of earlier research by Terman, whose research in 1998 revealed that bright light and high-density negative air ionization may both act as antidepressants in patients with seasonal affective disorder. They also paralleled the findings of Terman's 2005 paper on the effects of light and negative-ion therapies on non-seasonal chronic depression, which suggested that both treatments can relieve chronic depression just as well as they alleviate SAD. One of the most encouraging aspects of these results is the fact that these non-pharmaceutical interventions may help depressive patients avoid the side effects and contraindications common to antidepressant drugs.

As previously mentioned, the neurotransmitter serotonin plays a significant role in mood. Proper regulation of this chemical may be the key to beating depression, stress, and anxiety. Because serotonin has been associated with a calming effect, doctors typically rely on drugs known as selective serotonin reuptake inhibitors (SSRIs), which increase serotonin levels by limiting cellular reabsorption of this neurotransmitter, to treat these conditions. In doing so, they hope to encourage a state of tranquil sedation that might help the individual deal with any mental, emotional, or physiological stressors. Recent research, however, has been calling this approach into question. Contrary to previous belief, it appears that people with anxiety disorders may have levels of serotonin that are too high, not too low.

According to a study published in *JAMA Psychiatry,* researchers from the psychology department of Uppsala University were, in fact, able to show that individuals suffering from social phobia were making too much serotonin. More specifically, the research team, led by professors Mats Fredrikson and Tomas Furmark, found these elevated serotonin levels appearing in a part of the brain known as the amygdala, the brain's fear center. The more serotonin produced by a subject, the more anxious that subject became.

This study appears to mark a paradigm shift in our understanding of what is going on chemically in the brains of people suffering from anxiety. While scientists have known for some time that people with social anxiety also seem to have higher nerve activity in the amygdala, suggesting an overly sensitive fear center of the brain, these recent findings also point to excess serotonin as part of the mechanism that causes stress, anxiety, and depression. As stated by researcher Andreas Frick, "Serotonin can increase anxiety and not decrease it as was previously often assumed."

Television commercials advertising relaxation or meditation programs usually feature the idea of being outside in nature. That's no accident. Whether it's a yoga master meditating in the middle of a beach as birds are flying high above and the sun is setting over a divine landscape, or the soothing sounds of a waterfall emanating from a meditation soundtrack, these things have two main ideas in common: stress relief and nature. On a more personal note, you may have noticed that once you've worked for a long period of time and are due for a vacation, you try to find ways to keep yourself outside of buildings. The last thing you probably want to do is stay cooped up at your relatives' house or in a hotel room for the entirety of your vacation. No, you want to get out and explore, and breathe in some of the fresh air your body is craving. Time off, of course, can be very beneficial to your state of mind, regardless of negative-ion exposure. In light of this new interpretation of serotonin's role in mood, however, it would seem that the increased negative ions found outside the walls of your office play a large part in the way a vacation seems to decrease levels of stress, anxiety, and depression. (Some people have even called negative ions "vitamins of the air" due to their positive effects on the body and mind.)

While serotonin's true role in anxiety and other related mood disorders is only beginning to be revealed in mainstream research, a number of researchers have known about the power of negative-ion therapy in the battle against these difficult conditions for quite some time. Former Berkeley professor Dr. Albert P. Krueger dedicated much of his research to this subject, studying the effects of ions on both plants and animals for decades. His highly regarded work did much to move the subject of ion therapy from the fringe to a more respected place within the scientific community. On numerous occasions, Krueger saw that positive ions raised the serotonin levels of his animal test subjects, while negative ions lowered them. He also noted that these decreased serotonin concentrations were associated with many beneficial outcomes.

In 1967, American neuroscientist Allan H. Frey published a study in the *Journal of Comparative and Physiological Psychology* on the modification of emotional response by exposure to negative ions. He hypothesized that treatment with negative ions would cause a depletion of serotonin in the brain and predicted that mood would be affected by this therapy. His results were in accordance with his prediction. When animal subjects were treated with negative ions, their conditioned emotional responses to fear and anxiety were significantly reduced. Shortly thereafter, researcher Ronaldo Ucha Udabe and his fellow researchers also noted the positive effects of negative-ion therapy on a large number of patients with anxiety syndromes. Their sessions lasted from fifteen minutes to two hours, and the amount of treatments varied from ten to twenty. A vast majority of patients—about 80 percent of them—experienced relief from their disorders as a result of ion treatments.

In 1998, Russian scientists published the results of a study in which they exposed immobilized rats to negatively charged air ions. The researchers found that negative-ion treatment actually prevented the development of common symptoms of acute stress in all the subject animals, regardless of individual behavior type. Similarly, in 2001, Japanese researchers Ichiro Watanabe and Yukio Mano found that depressive scales and subjective feelings were improved through the use of negative-ion therapy. They even tested perspiration of the palm, which reflects sympathetic nerve function, and found that it decreased in the presence of negative ions, suggesting relief from stress and anxiety.

In 2013, a study published in *BMC Psychiatry* reviewed close to fifty years' worth of research papers on air ionization's possible effects on depression, anxiety, mood states, and feelings of mental well-being in humans. The researchers' thorough evaluation and analysis of these studies concluded that negative air ionization was strongly associated with lower rates of depression, particularly when high levels of negative ions were used. In this same year, two Italian researchers also published a review of the evidence base for the beneficial effects of negative air ions in improving mood disorders. Their analysis suggested that negative-ion therapy was generally effective in the treatment of mood disorders. According to the authors, "[t]he limitation in much of the literature on [negative-ion therapy] may have created the unsubstantiated impression that the treatment itself has limitations in terms of its efficacy. While pharmaceutical industry has devoted considerable resources for potential new antidepressant pharmacotherapies, there has not been a similarly endowed industry to support the development and testing of [negative-ion therapy]." Although the amount of clinical research being done on this subject has been growing, "there remain[s] a substantial gap in mental health services to translate state-of-the-art treatments and incorporate them into mainstream practice."

Japanese automobile manufacturer Toyota, however, has been researching negative ions for years. In one study from 2002, Toyota commissioned its research and development team to conduct an investigation into the effects of negative ions on drivers' mental stress and fatigue. The study, which was led by Dr. Kiyomi Sakakibara, set up two different driving simulators. Test subjects' stress and fatigue were monitored through sensory evaluations, driving performance, and adrenaline in their urine, which is a biochemical indicator of stress and fatigue.

In one driving simulator, six male subjects were told to drive as perfectly as possible on a round course, maintaining a steady high speed for fifty minutes. For the second driving simulator, fourteen male subjects were asked to drive at a much slower speed for sixty minutes, but they also needed to push certain buttons as fast as possible once one of three LEDs lit up. Both groups repeated their tasks twice—once with natural air (which was used as a control) and again with negative-ion exposure numbering close to 10,000 ions/cm^3, matching the ion output of a waterfall. The first group showed no difference in sensory evaluations (which were visual measurements), but much less adrenaline was found in their urine after the negative-ion conditions. The second group also showed no visually apparent differences in stress, but had smaller adrenaline levels in the urine after the negative-ion exposure as well. Additionally, the second group's missed button presses were reduced by 57 percent. The study's results also concluded that negative ions can improve a driver's cognitive performance. (See Cognitive Performance on page 47.) Intrigued by these results, Toyota continued its negative-ion research.

Another study was authored by Dr. Hideo Nakane in 2003 and focused exclusively on negative ions and the effect they might have on stress at a biological level. For the study, Dr. Nakane had twelve males participate in a classic psychology demonstration called the Stroop test. This test causes interference in reaction time by displaying names of colors printed in entirely different colors. For example, the word "green" might be printed in red, or the word "blue" might be printed in yellow. This causes people to take a longer time to name the color, and makes them more prone to error.

The subjects were divided into three groups, and all underwent three different experimental conditions: exposure to natural air, exposure to negative ions, and exposure to negative ions and fragrances. Each experiment began with a thirty-minute rest interval followed by the Stroop test for sixty minutes and concluded with another thirty minutes of rest. To measure stress, the research team collected saliva samples before the Stroop test, during it, and afterwards, with each round of exposure, as saliva produces a chemical known as chromogranin A (CgA) during times of stress. Results of these experiments showed that in the group that was not exposed to negative ions, levels of CgA continued to increase well into the Stroop task, while the group that received negative ions had very small, stable levels throughout the whole test.

It was revealed in 2012 that the Toyota Camry would come equipped with ionic technology, which would serve to enhance the car's air conditioning system and fill the cabin "with refreshing air characterized by an ultimately balanced ratio of positive and negative ions."

Witches' Winds Can Still Cast an Ugly Spell

According to the proverb, it's an ill wind that blows no one any good. For centuries, wherever warm, dry, harsh winds are common, tales of unhappiness have been associated with them, from folktales and legends to religious stories. These stories, however, may share a common factual basis. Known as witches' winds, these winds have many different names throughout the world. In the Middle East, this type of wind is called khamsin. Its Hebrew name is sharav. In Germany it is called a föhn wind, which roughly translates to "hairdryer." In the western United States, we call them the Santa Ana winds.

Regardless of their various names, these problematic winds are said to bring with them ailments and troublesome psychological changes. Residents who live in areas affected by these rough winds often report severe headaches, depression, carelessness, fever, or various other negative symptoms. There have even been reports of an association between witches' winds and increases in suicide and attempted suicide rates. For example, a study conducted at the Ludwig Maximilian University of Munich in Germany found that suicide and accidents increased by 10 percent during föhn winds in Central Europe. Humans have always been sensitive to atmospheric changes before, during, and after a storm, and this idea is reflected in everyday expressions such as "feeling under the weather" and feeling a storm "in your bones."

Many of the countries that experience these winds are aware of their effects but can do little to prevent them. The Swiss have previously blamed these winds for suicides, murders, car accidents, and domestic violence. In Germany, most notably in the Munich area, surgeons postpone surgeries if this type of wind has been forecast.

COGNITIVE PERFORMANCE

As noted in the research undertaken by Toyota in 2002, negative-ion exposure can increase cognitive performance. Years before this publication, however, researchers R.A. Duffee and R.H. Koontz were investigating ions and witnessing similar results. In 1965, they published a study in *Psychophysiology* that tested the effects of negatively ionized air on the cognitive functioning of rats. The study found that the rats' abilities to navigate a water maze improved by an average of 350 percent with negative-ion exposure, which suggested a significant boost in cognitive ability. Moreover, the performances of the older rats living in a negatively ionized atmosphere showed even more improvement.

In 1974, twenty subjects were exposed to negative ions and monitored by electroencephalogram (EEG), which records the electrical activity of the brain. Negative-ion therapy had measurable effects on brainwave patterns, and the subjective findings of the study's subjects included alertness and improvement in working capacity. A few years later, *Ergonomics* published a study that measured the effects of both negative and positive ions on the performance of psychomotor tasks and noted an association between negative-ion exposure and increased ability.

Robert A. Baron conducted a number of experiments with negative ions during the 1980s. In one experiment, male and female subjects worked on three different tasks— proofreading, memory span, word finding—in the presence of low, moderate, or high concentrations of negative ions. Results suggested that moderate amounts of these ions improved the males' performance on two of these tasks (proofreading and memory span). In another experiment, male and female subjects performed two additional tasks—copying a letter and making a decision—in the presence of low, moderate, or high concentrations of negative ions in the air. For both sexes, letter-copying ability increased significantly in the face of rising ion levels. In terms of decision making, the male subjects of this research displayed a tendency to select initially preferred alternatives when exposed to moderate amounts of negative ions. Baron's published study of these experiments showed that negative ions have the potential to boost cognitive performance. Moreover, this notable conclusion has actually been bolstered by the reports of a number of other researchers over the past few decades.

ATHLETIC PERFORMANCE

Just as negative ions may be used to elevate cognitive performance, they may also be used to improve athletic performance. Russian scientist A. A. Minkh analyzed the performance levels of Olympic athletes in different negative-ion conditions and observed that the group of athletes that trained and lived in areas with high concentrations of negative ions in the air also displayed vast improvements in performance as compared to the control group. In addition, Minkh's work revealed that negative-ion exposure led to faster reflexes in his subjects. Ultimately, Russian research has shown that athletes who take advantage of negative ions during training benefit from significant improvements in reaction time, balance, and endurance. Similarly, a study published in 1965, only a few years after Minkh's aforementioned work, showed a significant improvement in athletic performance in sportsmen treated with negative-ion therapy. It would seem that negative ions may be an easy way to stop the use of illegal performance-enhancing drugs by athletes.

CARDIOVASCULAR HEALTH

High levels of cholesterol in the blood (hypercholesterolemia) have been strongly linked to cardiovascular disease, as they result in atherosclerosis, otherwise known as hardening of the arteries. Although pharmaceutical companies have been treating this problem with cholesterol-lowering drugs for years, the use of negative ions to remedy this issue in a more natural way has shown promise for decades. As early as 1965, research has shown that negative ions have the ability to reduce blood cholesterol levels.

In 1975, young athletes treated with negative ions displayed increases in cardiovascular and respiratory adaptations to physical effort. The pulse, blood pressure, and respiration frequency of each athlete returned to normal levels sooner than expected. Around this same time, Russian scientist F.G. Portnov was also looking into the effects of negative-ion therapy. He found that exposure to negative ions demonstrated an ability to dilate blood vessels, known as vasodilation. When

Diabetics and the Elderly

Anyone exposed to air pollution is at risk for cardiovascular problems, but diabetics and the elderly are even more prone to heart damage. A study in *Epidemiology* closely examined almost a decade's worth of medical records from four major cities (Chicago, Detroit, Seattle, and Pittsburgh) and found that diabetics were twice as likely as non-diabetics to be admitted to hospital with cardiovascular issues due to air pollution. Additionally, they also found that elderly patients aged seventy-five or over faced a much higher risk of cardiovascular damage from airborne pollutants.

blood vessels relax and dilate, blood pressure lowers, as does stress on the cardiovascular system. (In addition, vasodilation may relieve migraines as well, as explained on page 36.) This mechanism was described in a 1985 study published in *Life Sciences*, which showed that 5-hydroxytryptophan, a precursor of serotonin, lowered blood pressure in a dose-dependent manner and in direct relation to the production of brain serotonin. It is clear that serotonin has a role in blood pressure regulation. The ability of negative ions to regulate serotonin levels, therefore, makes them a powerful agent in cardiovascular health.

In 2000, Dr. Yamada and Dr. Chino published a paper that described a study in which eight-week-old mice were fed high-cholesterol food for six days. One group of mice was exposed to negative ions and one group was not. The red blood cells of the negative-ion group displayed a separation and smoothness, while the red blood cells of the untreated group did not, suggesting beneficial cardiovascular outcomes in association with negative-ion therapy for individuals dealing with high cholesterol.

FREE RADICALS

Free radicals are atoms or groups of atoms with unpaired electrons. Because electrons like to exist in pairs, free radicals try to steal electrons from other molecules in order to even out their odd number. In the process, these highly reactive substances can start unwanted chain reactions of free-radical formation in the body. The main threat in this scenario is the terrible damage free radicals can do to important cellular components, including DNA. This damage may cause cells to function poorly and possibly even lead to increased rates of aging and a variety of problematic health conditions.

Although free radicals can harm cells, there are nevertheless an essential part of life and are constantly being created by the body. They can be formed in a number of ways, but perhaps the most common of free radicals, known as the reactive oxygen species (ROS), is made simply through the normal process of metabolism. As a counterbalance to the harmful aspects of free radicals, the body has a defense system of protective substances known as antioxidants. Antioxidants play a key role in the prevention of cellular damage, as they have the ability to neutralize free radicals and terminate the previously mentioned chain reactions before they lead to unwanted outcomes. Although the body naturally produces its own antioxidants, these helpful molecules may also be attained through diet. Vitamin antioxidants include vitamin E, beta-carotene, and vitamin C, all of which may be found in certain foods.

Some studies show that a diet rich in fruits and vegetables can lower rates of many diseases. It is generally thought that the antioxidants in these foods are responsible for their protective properties, as many fruits and vegetables are high in antioxidant vitamins and minerals. Research, however, is ongoing, and thus far inconclusive, as to whether antioxidant supplementation can be of use against sickness.

In relation to the important antioxidant superoxide dismutase (SOD), the effects of negative-ion therapy were studied in rat, bovine, man, and duck subjects. After being treated with negative ions (mostly superoxide) from an ion generator, subjects of the study displayed markers of increased levels of superoxide dismutase. In other words, researchers found that exposure to negative ions raised levels of the protective antioxidant superoxide dismutase. The authors of this study stated, "The stimulation of SOD activity by [negative air ions] NAI found in our experiments allows the understanding of the broad beneficial effects of [negative air ions] NAI." Negative ions, therefore, may have a role to play in protecting cells from damage caused by free radicals as well as the health issues associated with it.

SEROTONIN IRRITATION SYNDROME (SIS)

A number of pharmaceuticals, natural herbs, and amino acids can affect serotonin levels. The most obvious pharmaceutical examples are antidepressants known as selective serotonin reuptake inhibitors, or SSRIs. These drugs limit the reabsorption of serotonin into the cell, thereby increasing the amount of this neurotransmitter available to bind to its receptor. While the efficacy and safety of these drugs continue to be in dispute, they remain the most popular type of treatment prescribed by doctors for depression. Any substance that boosts serotonin's availability in the body, whether alone or in combination with other drugs or natural supplements that affect serotonin, may lead to dangerously high levels of this neurotransmitter. Excessive amounts of serotonin can result in a number of symptoms—some mild, some fatal—the entire spectrum of which is called serotonin irritation syndrome (SIS).

A mild case of serotonin irritation syndrome may cause an individual to exhibit troublesome signs such as increased heart rate, dilated pupils, twitching, sweating, and overactive reflexes (hyperreflexia). A moderate case may result in high blood pressure, elevated body temperature, agitation, and insomnia. Finally, a severe case may lead to terrible outcomes such as shock due to increased heart rate and blood pressure, seizures, renal failure, and disseminated intravascular coagulation, which refers to the formation of blood clots in the body's small blood vessels.

Serotonin irritation syndrome typically has a rapid onset and may be misdiagnosed as anxiety or a neurological disorder if symptoms are mild. Generally, SIS is treated through discontinuation of the drugs that lead to excessive serotonin in the body. Although SIS is most often the result of excessive serotonin caused by a combination of certain pharmaceuticals or the use of recreational drugs, some researchers are pointing to positive ions as a potential culprit. Positive ions have displayed the ability to elevate serotonin production when they significantly outnumber negative ions in the air. It would stand to reason that an environment high in positive ions would lead to SIS. If so, negative ions, which seem to lower serotonin production, may be an ideal therapy for this syndrome.

Research conducted by A.P. Krueger and colleagues and published in the *International Journal of Biometeorology* in 1968 showed that positive ions raised blood levels of serotonin in the mouse subject and negative ions decreased them. In 1979, Krueger hypothesized that positive ions raised serotonin and negative ions lowered serotonin due to their effects on monoamine oxidases (MAOs). According to Krueger, it was the stimulation of MAOs via negative-ion therapy that resulted in elevated serotonin, while the inhibition of this same family of enzymes via positive-ion exposure decreased levels of serotonin in the body. Furthermore, a study published in *Science* in 1980 found that animal subjects left in an environment rich in negative ions for twenty days had lower serotonin levels than those placed outside this exposure. The fact is that much research over the few decades has concluded that levels of negative ions are inversely related to serotonin levels. Just as sunlight disrupts sleep cycles by suppressing production of the hormone melatonin, negative ions suppress serotonin production. If the air is depleted of negative ions, an increase in serotonin follows.

F.G. Sulman published a study in the *Upsala Journal of Medical Sciences* on the subject of weather-induced migraines and headaches. It stated that "the electrical charges (positive ionisation and sferics) engendered by every incoming weather front produce a release of serotonin." Essentially, certain changes in weather and their resultant effects on serotonin levels could lead to the onset of a group of symptoms known as serotonin irritation syndrome. According to the study, weather disturbances were behind the migraines and headaches of 20 to 30 percent of the population, but these conditions could be remedied with "appropriate treatment." In other research, Sulman noted that serotonin irritation syndrome was caused by conditions that occur during annual wind storms such as the Sirocco, sharav, and Santa Ana winds. These winds lead to positive ionization of the air, which results in SIS. Appropriately, Sulman also suggested treatment options for this problem, including the addition of negative ions to the environments of those affected by weather-related SIS, which could lower serotonin in sufferers and eliminate their migraines and headaches.

In light of this description of serotonin irritation syndrome, it is remarkable how many people may be helped by an increase in negative ions in the air. According to a 1986 research paper, almost one-third of the population appears to be particularly sensitive to negative-ion depletion, making them very susceptible to serotonin irritation syndrome. So many people may be dealing with SIS unknowingly, experiencing symptoms that mimic other health conditions, lead to misdiagnoses, and result in ineffective treatments that may have unwanted side effects. The time to bring SIS into mainstream medical understanding seems far overdue, and the time to take advantage of negative-ion therapy to remedy this syndrome is undoubtedly now.

SLEEP

One major problem that continues to increase in the United States is sleep disorders. According to the National Sleep Foundation, approximately 62 percent of all Americans have trouble sleeping at least a few times per week, and around 30 percent of all adults (about 70 million people) have insomnia each year. According to the Centers for Disease Control (CDC), this troubling trend is only growing in numbers. The dangers of sleep deprivation go beyond just having a bad day at work. The CDC currently recognizes insufficient sleep as a public health epidemic because it has been linked to motor vehicle crashes, industrial disasters, and medical errors. Close to 5 percent of the American population has fallen asleep or dozed off momentarily while behind the wheel during the last month, resulting in more than 42,000 car crashes each year, with 1,550 of those crashes resulting in fatalities.

Although the neurotransmitter serotonin has been associated with a calming effect in regard to mood, countless studies now show that when serotonin levels are too high, serotonin irritation syndrome can soon follow, resulting in symptoms such as agitation, insomnia, and even seizures. It is no wonder research has shown that exposure to negative ions, which lower serotonin, may promote healthy sleep patterns.

This idea is backed up by a 1987 study published in *Biological Psychiatry,* which exposed eight manic-depressive patients to negative ions to treat their symptoms. Of the eight, seven subjects experienced improved sleep from lowered serotonin levels. In 1991, research showed that overproduction of serotonin could cause sleeplessness and nightmares. When a negative-ion generator was used to treat a group of subjects suffering from these results of too much serotonin, most members became better able to sleep.

To better understand the effects negative ions can have on sleep, it is important to take a look at the subject of circadian rhythms. Essentially, circadian rhythms are biological fluctuations that follow an approximately twenty-four-hour cycle. These changes occur in practically all living things, including animals, plants, and a large number of microbes, and are crucial to sleep patterns and eating patterns. They are regulated by groups of interacting molecules throughout the body known as "biological clocks." These biological clocks are coordinated by a "master clock" made up of small nuclei in the middle of the brain called the suprachiasmatic nuclei, or SCN. Light and darkness in the environment play major roles in setting the body's master clock, and thus its circadian rhythms. The most obvious example of these time cues is sunlight, which is the reason some blind people have problems with their sleep. Other factors that affect the SCN include exercise, hormones, and medications.

In order to be healthy, the circadian rhythms need to act in concert with each other, playing their roles at the appropriate times. For example, body temperature rises during the last hours of sleep prior to waking up and decreases when the time for sleep begins at night. (Most people also experience a drop in body temperature in the mid to late afternoon, which may be related to a sleepy feeling commonly felt at this time of day.) Simply put, internal "clocks" regulate circadian rhythms, which dip and rise throughout the day, creating feelings of sleepiness and wakefulness. Of course, if you have had enough sleep overnight, the sleepiness experienced during circadian dips should be less severe.

Circadian rhythms actually change throughout a person's lifetime. During adolescence, most teens experience a shift in their sleep phases, which makes them feel more alert later at night. As a result, during this period it becomes harder to fall asleep at a reasonable hour. Unfortunately, early school start times do not mesh well with a teenager's circadian rhythms and often leads to sleep deprivation.

In 1993, researchers Reilly and Stevenson exposed male subjects to negative ions and measured physiological responses, including body temperature, heart rate, and respiration while at rest and during exercise. Negative ions were found to significantly improve all physiological states, particularly during rest. Most important was "Results confirm that negative air ions are biologically active and that they do affect the body's circadian rhythmicity."

As sleep is the time during which the body's cells are repaired and regenerated, any therapy that might regulate circadian rhythms and improve sleep patterns should be further investigated. The importance of sleep cannot be overstated.

WEIGHT LOSS

There are many detoxification diets (more often called "detox diets") that claim to help cleanse your body and rid it of any impurities that may have accumulated over time. But what good is a cleaner body if the mind remains unchanged? Bad habits will resume, lifestyle changes will be temporary, and the diet will become just another failed attempt at getting and staying healthy, akin to the notoriously difficult New Year's resolution of losing weight.

Countless studies have shown that high stress and anxiety levels are linked to weight gain, which could lead to health complications such as an increased risk of stroke, high blood pressure, and diabetes, to name just a few. This is because stress affects a person both physically and emotionally. If you are going through major life events or even simply having a rough day, you may find yourself snacking more throughout the day and overeating during meals. Worse still, during times of stress, your body may crave "comfort food," which is typically high-calorie food loaded with sugar or fat, including fried food, chocolate, ice cream, and pasta.

Carbohydrates increase levels of serotonin, which is why your body yearns for carbs during times of duress. This mood elevation is temporary, however, and is usually followed by a crash. Although they might provide temporary relief, excess carbs and the associated weight gain are not worth it. Exposure to large numbers of negative ions can lower your stress by regulating the neurotransmitter serotonin. It can also lower anxiety by reducing levels of cortisol, a stress-related hormone that has been linked to increased fat in the abdomen.

In addition to a sound diet and proper exercise, it is important to eliminate any other factors that may contribute to weight gain and poor eating habits. By greatly decreasing unwanted stress and anxiety through negative-ion exposure, you are removing one more obstacle on the road to the state of health you desire.

As a side note, the negative ions found in fresh air keep your body feeling great, and this positive association with nature can help encourage you to spend more time outdoors, resulting in increased physical activity and weight loss. Spending upwards of forty-five minutes on a treadmill or stationary bicycle in a gym packed with sweaty bodies and stale, recirculated air just doesn't sound as appealing as spending the same amount of time jogging or riding a bicycle through a scenic bike path in a cool breeze, does it? Our bodies are designed to benefit most from being outside in a natural environment, not from sitting in a cramped cubicle hunched over a computer for eight to ten hours a day while being constantly bombarded by excessive amounts of air pollution and positive ions.

CONCLUSION

The power of negative and positive ions can have a great degree of influence on a number of the body's internal systems as well as behavior and attitude. Environments with excessive levels of positive ions can have detrimental effects on a whole host of issues, including mood, immune system function, cognitive performance, athletic performance, cardiovascular health, sleep patterns, and more. To make things worse, these health conditions often overlap, perpetuating each other and furthering negative outcomes. For example, high levels of positive ions can cause anxiety and other mood disorders, which can lead to problems with sleep. A lack of sleep can then make anxiety and other mood disorders worse. It's a vicious circle that should be stopped before it takes shape.

Research suggests that negative ions can have a wide variety of potential benefits in regard to these health problems. The only way to see if you can improve your own health condition, however, is to expose yourself to negative ions. The good thing is that negative-ion therapy is now available in a few different forms. The following chapter provides a list of devices that can help you find the right treatment for you.

4

Negative-Ion Devices

Now that you are familiar with the health benefits associated with negative ions and recognize the danger of overexposure to positive ions, it is time to experience some of the positive effects of negative ions for yourself. Over the last decade, a number of products have been designed to produce higher levels of negative ions in the air. These amounts are measured in cubic centimeters, or cm^3 (sometimes cc or ccm), which refer to the concentration of ions in one cubic centimeter of space.

For normal human function, an optimal level is 1,000 negative ions per cubic centimeter, or 1,000 negative ions/cm^3. Research suggests that amounts above 1,000 negative ions/cm^3 start to have therapeutic effects, while dosages of 10,000 negative ions/cm^3 and above seem to be ideal in providing relief from many health conditions. In this chapter, you will find methods of naturally receiving negative ions as well as descriptions of the most affordable and conveniently designed negative-ion generators on the market.

NATURALLY OCCURRING NEGATIVE IONS

As you are now aware, high concentrations of both positive ions and negative ions may be found in different locations throughout nature and even at different times. For example, you may experience a headache or feel tense right before a severe thunderstorm occurs. After the storm has ended, the air seems to refresh you and your headache passes. Coincidentally, there is an enormous amount of positive ions generated before a storm, while the air after a storm has a notably high level of negative ions. While negative ions may be found in many places throughout the great outdoors, the best natural sources have moving water that crashes against surfaces.

The positive and negative ions found in our surroundings can vary in number depending on a variety of factors, including temperature, humidity, and air circulation. A car with its windows closed contains around 15 negative ions/cm^3. Turn the air conditioner on, and that number can drop to 1 negative ion/cm^3. An average room contains approximately 150 negative ions/cm^3. A well-insulated office building has about 50 negative ions/cm^3, which is around the same amount as the outdoor air of a polluted city. Outdoor air in cities with low pollution contains around 300 to 400 negative ions/cm^3. Stand near a creek or river and you could be exposed to approximately 600 negative ions/cm^3. Large fountains can produce upwards of 1,000 negative ions/cm^3, while forests contain more than 3,000 negative ions/cm^3. Close to the shore of a beach contains about 4,000 negative ions/cm^3, depending on wave strength and wind. Small waterfalls can produce between 5,000 and 10,000 negative ions/cm^3, while large waterfalls can produce between 10,000 and 50,000 negative ions/cm^3. Niagara Falls and similarly sized waterfalls can produce 100,000 negative ions/cm^3.

As you can see, amounts of negative ions can vary widely based on many factors. It is also important to understand that positive and negative ions exist together in most environments. As you will find, particular environments can greatly influence your well-being both physically and mentally, in both good ways and bad. The key is to limiting your exposure to high levels of positive ions and spend more time in areas rich in negative ions, as doing so may have a significant effect on your health. You may use the chart below as a quick guide to the average concentrations of negative ions found in various environments.

AVERAGE CONCENTRATION OF NEGATIVE IONS BY ENVIRONMENT

Environment	Negative Ions/cm^3
Air-conditioned Indoors	0–100
Roads with Heavy Traffic	100–300
Well-ventilated Home	500
Riverside	600
Countryside	1,000
Large Fountain	1,000
Forest	3,000
Beach	4,000
Small Waterfall	5,000–10,000
Large Waterfall	10,000–50,000
Niagara Falls	100,000

While you may not be able to visit Niagara Falls on a regular basis, the information provided by this chart certainly suggests taking a walk in nature more often. These outdoor environments can be refreshing not only thanks to their beauty but also because of the elevated concentrations of negative ions they provide.

MAN-MADE NEGATIVE IONS

If you lead a busy lifestyle, as so many Americans do, it is perfectly understandable that you might not be able to spend several hours a day in the middle of a serene landscape by a babbling brook or dazzling waterfall. Luckily, there are several solutions. Two of the most common means to become exposed to negative ions are man-made negative ion generators and wearable bands. In the following sections, you will learn about the major differences between these two methods of exposure, what to look for when purchasing each type, and which one might be the best choice for you to make when it comes to supplying your body with the negative ions it needs.

Negative-Ion Air Purifiers

When it comes to negative-ion generators, the choices are vast. These machines are often called air ionizers in retail stores and are available in many different sizes and at many different price points. Finding one that is best for your situation and budget can mean the difference between fully experiencing the benefits of negative ions and not feeling anything at all.

Air ionizers can work in several ways, but one of the most common methods of generating negative ions is by charging nearby air molecules through high voltage. Inside each generator there is a grounded conductor and an electrode that attracts positive ions. Once the positively charged ions make their way into the filter of the device, these particles cling to the grounded surface, at which point newly negatively charged atoms float back into the air.

Another type of negative-ion generator is believed by many to be the most effective at generating sufficient levels of negative ions. It involves using the same high voltage as the sort previously mentioned, but this time current is applied to the sharp, microscopic points of an "ion emitter." Electricity causes electrons to build up on these sharp points. After a certain point, these electrons are ejected from the ion emitter's tips into the air. Once in the air, these electrons find the closest oxygen molecule and cling to it, giving it a negative charge. As mentioned at the outset of this book, once a molecule gains more electrons than protons, it becomes a negative ion.

Small, portable ion generators exist that look similar in design to scented-oil warmers. These tiny ionizers are best used for small-scale needs, such as cleaning the air of your personal office or neutralizing the positive ions of your TV screen at home. Prices typically range between $15 and $30. These machines do not produce nearly enough negative ions to cover a whole room, so place them as close to your body as possible. For air ionizers that can cover whole rooms, expect to pay anywhere from $150 to $400. Unlike the small generators, most medium-sized negative-ion generators are meant to be run twenty-four hours a day and do not have an off switch, but are usually energy-efficient machines that are self-cleaning, easy to maintain, and quiet.

Directions for use vary with each manufacturer, but usually you'll want to avoid placing these devices on bookcases or shelves, as doing so may accidentally trap the negative ions within that enclosed space. Instead, place it on the floor or front edge of a table and keep it within three to five feet of your head.

Whole-house units do exist, but they can cost anywhere from $1,000 to a staggering $5,000 or more. These units need to be periodically cleaned, tend to run a little louder than other ionizers, and are more difficult to find.

An ion generator can produce between 1,000 and 10,000 negative ions per cubic centimeter, and some even claim to generate an astonishing 1,000,000 negative ions/cm^3. Recall that 1,000 negative ions/cm^3 is the amount required for normal human health, but if you're looking for a therapeutic dosage, between 1,000 negative ions/cm^3 and 10,000 negative ions/cm^3 is the adequate level. Refer to each manufacturer for exact numbers, but keep in mind that these levels can vary greatly depending on several factors, including humidity and circulation.

Although the United States is beginning to bring negative-ion generators into the mainstream, other countries such as Japan have been embracing this technology for years. In Japan, negative-ion generators may be found in many household appliances and gadgets, including refrigerators, air conditioners, washing machines, and toothbrushes. The Taiwanese computer manufacturer company ASUS even includes an integrated negative-ion generator in some of its laptops. As this technology is still relatively unknown in the United States, it is very important to verify that the negative-ion generator you are interested in buying does not produce harmful ozone, which, unfortunately, many of these devices do. Ozone is a toxic gas, which, when inhaled, can damage the lungs. According to the United States Environmental Protection Agency (EPA), "[r]elatively low amounts can cause chest pain, coughing, shortness of breath, and throat irritation. Ozone may also worsen chronic respiratory diseases such as asthma and compromise the ability of the body to fight respiratory infections."

Negative-Ion Bands

Air ionizers are a great way to produce negative ions in the comfort of your own home and at the office, but what if you are on the go and can't be at either of those places? The solution may be a negative-ion band, often simply called an ion band, or ion bracelet. Although wearing an ion band may help you benefit from negative ions while on the move, these devices are much more controversial than the negative-ion generators described earlier, as they are not connected to any electric current and thus have to rely on self-generated forces to produce the benefits associated with negative ions.

Ion bracelets are essentially wristbands that contain specific chemical elements, minerals, or combinations of certain naturally occurring substances. The most prevalent constituent of negative-ion bands is tourmaline, although sometimes they may also include amethyst or germanium, which have properties similar to tourmaline, or titanium, which claims to maximize performance of negative ion-generating materials such as tourmaline. (There are also some indications that titanium contains properties that may help relax muscles and make the wearer feel more refreshed.) Tourmaline and these other possible components are typically embedded in silicone rubber, which is commonly what these bands look and feel like, although sometimes they are placed in a bracelet of stainless steel or titanium.

In addition to the capacity of tourmaline to generate negative ions, germanium, amethyst, and tourmaline seem to emit far-infrared radiation, which is said to have certain therapeutic properties.

Far infrared (FIR) forms the section of the electromagnetic spectrum just below visible light. Far-infrared rays, however,

Negative Ions versus Ozone

In an effort to jump on the bandwagon, some companies have machines that are sold as "ion generators" but, in reality, are ozone generators. It is important to know that there is a huge difference between ozone and negative ions. First, their compositions are entirely different. Ozone (O_3) is a molecule made up of three oxygen atoms, as opposed to the oxygen we breathe, which contains only two. Negative ions, however, are molecules that simply possess an extra electron. Negative ions are extremely beneficial to the body and mind, while ozone can cause damage to delicate body tissues such as the lungs and heart with prolonged exposure.

Negative-ion generators are meant to reduce the number of particulates in the air, making it cleaner, while ozone does not remove any particulates from the air. Ozone generators mislabeled as negative-ion generators are becoming so common now that the EPA released a lengthy and thorough report on the dangers of not properly researching air ionizers before purchasing one, stating exactly what ozone is and giving recommendations for alternatives to ozone generators.

Legitimate and properly labeled ozone generators exist, but their purpose is not to clean the air of dangerous particulates; it is to remove odors from the air. Negative ions clean the air but are not effective at removing odors. Ozone is highly effective at removing even the strongest odor. An ozone generator may be purchased purely for odor control as long as it is used with caution.

are not to be confused with ultraviolet rays, or UV rays, which are known to be potentially harmful to the body. An easy way to experience far-infrared radiation would be to apply sunscreen and lie out in the sun. Have you ever wondered why you still feel heat from the sun's radiation when you are wearing sunblock? The answer is far-infrared radiation, which penetrates the skin even when dangerous UV rays are being denied absorption by sunscreen.

The human body itself radiates in the far-infrared range at a wavelength of approximately 9 micrometers, or microns. (These far-infrared rays emitted by the body may account for the origin of the Chinese idea of "chi," which refers to the body's natural life force and is a central principle in traditional Chinese medicine.) Certain chemical elements, such as germanium, give off far-infrared radiation at wavelengths close to or exactly that of the human body. When these wavelengths match in frequency, a resonance is created with the body's water molecules. Resonance refers to the tendency of a system to increase its amplitude of oscillation when exposed to an outside force with an equal or almost identical natural frequency. In other words, far-infrared radiation released at the same frequency of the body's far-infrared radiation excites water molecules and, as a result, may improve blood circulation. As approximately 70 percent of the body is made up of water, the effects of this resonance may be notable, potentially rejuvenating organs throughout the body.

There are many manufacturers of negative-ion bands, and some of the larger companies include Energy Armor, Ionic Balance, and Fusion Ionz. Prices generally range from $15 to about $40, but some bracelets can reach or exceed $100. The majority of negative-ion ion bands produce between 1,500 and 4,000 negative ions/cm^3, depending on the elements they contain, although negative-ion companies are always making efforts to increase output levels of future products. Typically, a negative-ion band's effectiveness should far outlast its user, but it is always wise to check the production description of any bracelet you may be considering to find out its purported shelf life, so to speak. While negative-ion bands may produce fewer negative ions than do negative-ion air purifiers, there is a theory that suggests a greater number of negative ions actually reach and affect your body when generated by a negative-ion bracelet, so the difference between the levels of negative ions experienced from a negative-ion generator and those from a negative-ion band may not be so significant. In addition, many negative-ion ion bands are waterproof, and some even include functional watches.

Tourmaline

If you have been looking into buying a negative-ion wristband, you have surely seen tourmaline being used as a main component. This is because tourmaline is one of only a handful of substances that seem to have the capacity to produce both negative ions and far-infrared rays. In fact, this crystalline mineral is known by many for its purported ability to cleanse and detoxify the body, aid in fat loss, reduce water retention, and improve blood circulation. Taken from the Sinhalese term "tura mali," tourmaline roughly translates to "stone mixed with vibrant colors." This semiprecious stone is compounded with a number of chemical elements, the amounts of which may vary from stone to stone. These variations cause tourmaline to be found in a number of different colors, including vibrant shades of yellow, green, blue, red, and black. Many claim that there are no two tourmaline gemstones in the world with exactly the same coloration. This gemstone is hugely popular in Japan, where many Japanese baseball players may be seen wearing it both on and off the field.

As previously stated, negative-ion bracelets claim to emit negative ions and yet, unlike the machines that generate ions, do not use an external power supply to do so. This notion has caused them to come under particular scrutiny. Where tourmaline is concerned, however, there may be a satisfactory response to this criticism. From a scientific standpoint, tourmaline is known to generate a weak electric current. This naturally mild charge of this gemstone may be behind its suggested healthful properties.

Tourmaline is what is known as a piezoelectric stone, which means it can generate an electric charge when mechanical stress is applied to its surface. A number of products, in fact, rely on the piezoelectric effect of various ceramics, gemstones, and even bone—microphones, quartz watches, and inkjet printers are but a few of them. It has even been said that Benjamin Franklin, the inventor of the lightning rod, was familiar with tourmaline and used a tourmaline stone in some of his experiments. In 1880, French physicist Pierre Curie (husband of Marie Curie), along with his brother Jacques, discovered that electricity could be generated by putting pressure on certain materials, including tourmaline. The term piezoelectricity, in fact, is derived from the Greek word "piezein," which means "squeeze." In addition to its piezoelectric properties, tourmaline is also pyroelectric, which means it is able to generate voltage when heated or cooled.

Research has shown that tourmaline also produces far-infrared radiation. This far-infrared radiation, along with its piezoelectric and pyroelectric capabilities, is thought to be sufficient to convert moisture from the air into negative ions. For these reasons, the proponents of tourmaline see this stone as the most natural and safe way to create negative ions.

A paper by Harvard University researchers addressed the use of a particular subdivision of the far-infrared waveband, which "has been observed in both *in vitro* and *in vivo* studies, to stimulate cells and tissue, and is considered a promising treatment modality for certain medical conditions." The authors stated that "the boron-silicate mineral, tourmaline (known as a gemstone in its crystalline form) when milled into fine powders also emits FI," and that "[p]reparations containing tourmaline powder have been applied to the skin with the aim of affecting the blood flow." Ultimately, the study remarked on the need for further investigation into FIR-emitting materials, noting that "the possible future applications are wide ranging."

A study published in the *Journal of Nanoscience and Nanotechnology* looked at very finely ground tourmaline and concluded that tourmaline superfine powder actually exhibited increased far-infrared emissions as the particle size decreased. Obviously, this research bodes well for those products that include very finely ground tourmaline as a component, as many negative-ion bands do.

While tourmaline's role in health improvement remains unclear and warrants further study, it is worth noting that "[c]ontrary to previous presumption, accumulated evidence indicates that far-infrared rays are biologically active." According to a 1989 study in the *International Journal of Biometeorology*, the majority of users of ceramic disks that emitted far-infrared radiation reported improvements in their health. Despite the fact that these evaluations were completely subjective, they remain worthy of consideration. These results may have been due to the far-infrared rays alone, or they may have occurred thanks to negative ions generated with the help of FIR. Although we do not yet know the exact mechanism through which tourmaline generates negative ions or its associated health benefits, it seems reasonable to assume that its FIR-emitting, piezoelectric, and pyroelectric properties may work together to turn atoms into negative ions and boost well-being.

Amethyst

Quartz is the second-most common mineral in the Earth's continental crust. Amethyst is the popular violet-colored version of quartz. Although amethyst is the rarest form of this mineral, it is nevertheless widely available around the world. The purple color of amethyst varies in shade from dark purple to lavender. Throughout history, this form of quartz has been used to treat a number of problems. It was even thought to combat drunkenness, which is why its name comes from the Ancient Greek words meaning "not intoxicated." Amethyst has also been considered therapeutic for hearing problems, sleep disorders, and even pain.

Like tourmaline, amethyst is believed to produce negative ions and give off far-infrared radiation. As such, this mineral is said to offer the same health benefits promised by tourmaline. These claims are supported by the fact that, like tourmaline, amethyst is piezoelectric. It, too, is capable of generating its own electrical current.

Germanium

Germanium is a chemical element. Like tourmaline, germanium is commonly found in ion bands. It was named after the country of Germany, where scientist Clemens Winkler discovered this element in 1886. It is a metalloid that is considered a semiconductor, which means it conducts electricity but does so not quite as well as a true metal. This important characteristic is what made it the material used in the world's first point-contact transistor, made by Bell Labs in the late 1940s. In addition, germanium allows infrared rays to pass through it. Because of this special property, many pieces of equipment that require infrared rays to pass through them are made using germanium.

Although much more study is warranted in this area, when it comes to ion bracelets, it would seem as though germanium's two most relevant properties are the way in which it may encourage far-infrared rays to benefit the body and its ability to reduce excessive levels of positive ions. In regard to the latter quality, the germanium atom has thirty-two electrons, and an electron configuration that places four of these electrons on its outermost shell. Germanium has been proven susceptible, however, to electron holes. An electron hole refers to an electron becoming excited into a higher state, which forces this electron to exit its position and leave a hole where one electron could exist in an atom. This process may be exhibited when germanium is met by a foreign substance that raises the temperature above 32 degrees Celsius. This rise in temperature causes one of the four electrons on the outermost shell to be ejected out of its orbit. This free electron may help neutralize a nearby positive ion, and if enough positive ions are neutralized, the ill effects of excessive positive-ion exposure may be alleviated. In terms of negative-ion bracelets that include germanium as an ingredient, when heated above 32 degrees Celsius by its proximity to the body, this known semiconductor should produce a significant amount of free electrons, which may have the capacity to mitigate positive-ion levels and thereby result in health benefits.

In addition to its free electrons, germanium possesses the ability to respond to infrared light in a rather unique way for a semiconductor, allowing it to pass through its structure. This characteristic is a major reason why so many ion bracelets include germanium in their components. The capacity to eliminate positive ions while also enabling far-infrared emissions to bring about healthful outcomes would seem to make germanium an ideal ingredient in a negative-ion band.

Top Five Bands by Negative-Ion Emission

Testing of a wide variety of negative-ion bands revealed the top five bands according to negative-ion emission. They were as follows:

1. Fusion IONZ
2. Ion Me
3. Ionic Balance
4. I-ONICS
5. LIFESTRENGTH

The COM SYSTEMS 3010 Pro Negative Ion Tester was used to measure the negative-ion production of each band and care was taken to avoid variance in results. Of course, as products improve over time, this list will surely change, so it is important to do your research before purchasing any negative-ion bracelet.

Which Is Best?

As mentioned, Japanese baseball players are known to wear black tape or black bracelets containing tourmaline or some combination of the typical constituents of negative-ion bands. In the United States, some MLB players and NFL players may be seen wearing similar necklaces or bracelets. It is difficult to say exactly which type of ion wristband will work best for you, but generally speaking, the best negative-ion wristband will usually include a combination of tourmaline, germanium, and titanium. When crushed up into particles, these three ingredients may result in a highly conductive wristband, as the germanium will allow far-infrared radiation to help activate tourmaline's negative-ion production as well as lead to other positive health outcomes. The benefits of all three minerals should compound, leaving you feeling much better if you've been sitting in an environment rich in positive ions for a period of time. While negative-ion wristbands may be slightly more controversial than negative-ion air purifiers, they do have the benefit of portability. You can wear a wristband throughout your day, while an air purifier is advantageous only if you are nearby one of these devices.

Of course, if you are interested in trying a negative-ion bracelet, you should approach this therapy with appropriate caution and understanding, particularly if you are suffering from a chronic illness. As is the case with any health product, it would be wise to consult with your doctor before using a negative-ion wristband. If you use any electrical medical device, such as a pacemaker, definitely consult your doctor before trying any negative-ion therapy.

CONCLUSION

When selecting a negative-ion product, always do your homework. You should take the time to understand the pros and cons of the equipment under consideration. Make sure the manufacturer stands behind its product. Don't be afraid to ask questions. While the Internet is a great resource, be aware that you may see some unbelievable claims on websites that have been designed simply to sell a product rather than to enlighten readers. The more you learn about the power of negative ions, the better decisions you will be able to make regarding negative-ion devices.

Conclusion

I have been lucky enough to work in the fields of pharmacy, herbal research, and nutrition for over fifty years. Over the course of my career, I have had the opportunity to see many of my books published in numerous languages around the world. What continues to motivate me is my love of educating people on simple, natural, noninvasive ways to produce optimal health. What I have found, however, time and time again, is that while I can offer direction in a book, a book is only the first step on the path to better health. The information I provide is useless if readers do not take the next steps.

Handing your well-being over to the healthcare system isn't always the appropriate answer. You should take as much responsibility for your own health as you can. If you are not feeling well, you may have the power to do something about it. In the case of a number of ailments, that power may be found in negative ions. With negative ions, there are no operations involved, no pills to take, and no problematic side effects to worry about. If this book has inspired you to increase your exposure to high levels of negative ions (and to avoid excessive levels of positive ions), then you may be on your way to good feelings. Once you bring more negative ions into your life, you may find your health problems begin to clear up or your chronic pain starts to disappear. These outcomes will mean you have finally discovered a natural way to heal your body and refresh your mind.

When it comes to the benefits of negative ions, I urge you to learn as much as you can, ask questions, and seek second or third opinions. Do not be afraid to become an active participant in your own well-being. I wish simply that you be well and remain healthy.

Resources

The following organizations make up the top five producers of negative-ion bands, as listed on page 75. Take your time to research any product claiming to emit negative ions, as not all are created equal.

Fusion IONZ
www.fusionpowerbandz.com
support@fusionionz.com
Founded by Matthew Ryncarz, who credits negative-ion technology for turning his life around, Fusion IONZ aims to bring the consumer good health through science and technology. The company subjects all its products to rigorous scientific testing in order to back up performance claims and ensure top-quality merchandise.

Ion Me
3187-C Airway Ave.
Costa Mesa, CA 92626
1-877-704-4667
www.ionme.com
info@ionme.com
Ion Me seeks to provide the highest quality negative-ion products on the market. Through its unique design and proprietary technology, Ion Me has become a top choice for professional athletes and people seeking a healthy lifestyle.

Ionic Balance
1 Carsegate Road North
Inverness
IV3 8DU
UK
www.ionic-balance.com
shop@ionic-balance.com
+44 1463 360 160
Based in the UK, Ionic Balance produces negative-ion wristbands, watches, braids, necklaces, and pet tags, all of which use a proprietary active formula of tourmaline and ten other components.

I-ONICS
1201-1202 Tower 2 China Hong Kong City,
33 Canton Road
Tsim Sha Tsui
Kowloon
Hong Kong
+852 2730 2626
www.i-onics.com

Based in China, I-ONICS works hard to make the best, most practical negative-ion bands available. They are so confident in their products that they offer a full thirty-day money-back guarantee.

LIFESTRENGTH
Kenex d.o.o.
Sela pri Dobovi 3 a
8257 Dobova
Slovenia
+386 7 49 66 960
www.lifestrength.si/en
info@lifestrength.si

LIFESTRENGTH uses an exclusive process that uniquely aggregates the beneficial properties of seven minerals and gemstones in one performance-enhancing and attractive bracelet. It offers a proprietary blend of minerals that create negative ions to counteract the overabundance of positively charged particles found in the modern world.

References

CHAPTER 2

Cheney, M. *Tesla: Man Out of Time.* New York, NY: Dorset Press, 1989.

Tesla, Nikola. "The Problem of Increasing Human Energy—With Special Reference to the Harnessing of the Sun's Energy." *The Century* (June 1900): Vol. LX, No. 2.

CHAPTER 3

Allergies and Asthma

Adar, S.D., Sheppard, L., Vedal, S., Polak, J.F., Sampson, P.D., Diez Roux, A.V., Budoff, M., Jacobs, D.R. Jr., Barr, R.G., Watson, K., and J.D. Kaufman. "Fine particulate air pollution and the progression of carotid intima-medial thickness: a prospective cohort study from the multi-ethnic study of atherosclerosis and air pollution." *PLoS Med* (2013): 10(4).

Asthma and Allergy Foundation of America (AAFA). www.aafa.org.

Gualtierotti, R., Solimene, U., and D. Tonoli. "Ionized air respiratory rehabilitation technics." *Minerva Medica* (1977): 68: 3383–3389.

Krueger, A.P. and R.F. Smith. "The effects of air ions of the living mammalian trachea. *J Gen Physiol* (Sep 1958): 20;42(1): 69–82.

Lipin, I., Gur, I., Amitai, Y., Amirav, I., and S. Godfrey. "Effect of positive ionisation of inspired air on the response of asthmatic children to exercise." *Thorax* (Aug 1984): 39(8): 594–596.

Mitchell, B.W., Buhr, R.J., Berrang, M.E., Bailey, J.S., and N.A. Cox. "Reducing airborne pathogens, dust and Salmonella transmission in experimental hatching cabinets using an electrostatic space charge system." *Poult Sci* (Jan 2002): 81(1): 49–55.

Palti, Y., De Nour, E., and A. Abrahamov. "The effect of atmospheric ions on the respiratory system of infants." *Pediatrics* (Sep 1966): 38(3): 405-11.

Pope, C.A. 3rd, Burnett, R.T., Thun, M.J., Calle, E.E., Krewski, D., Ito, K., and G.D. Thurston. "Lung cancer, cardiopulmonary mortality, and long-term exposure to fine particulate air pollution." *JAMA* (Mar 2002): 6; 287(9): 1132-41.

"Questions About Your Community: Indoor Air." *United States Environmental Protection Agency (EPA)*. www.epa.gov/region1/communities/indoorair.html.

Seo, K.H., Mitchell, B.W., Holt, P.S., and R.K. Gast. "Bactericidal effects of negative air ions on airborne and surface Salmonella enteritidis from an artificially generated aerosol." *J Food Prot* (Jan 2001): 64(1):113–6.

ADHD

Craig F. Garfield et al. "Trends in attention deficit hyperactivity disorder (ADHD) ambulatory diagnosis and medical treatment in the United States, 2000-2010." *Acad Pediatr* (Mar 2012): 12(2): 110–116.

Morton, L.L. and John R. Kershner. "Differential negative air ion effects on learning disabled and normal-achieving children." *International Journal of Biometeorology* (1990): 34(1): 35–41.

Morton, L.L. and John R. Kershner. "Negative air ionization improves memory and attention in learning-disabled and mentally retarded children." *Journal of Abnormal Child Psychology* (June 1984): 12(2): 353–365.

Terry, R. A., Harden, D.G., and A. M. Mayyasi. "Effects of negative air ions, noise, sex and age on maze learning in rats." *International Journal of Biometeorology* (June 1969): 13(1): 39–49.

Healing and the Immune System

Benko, G. "Analyse du mécanisme d'action des ions atmosphériques de forte concentration, de polarité différente, sur des animaux expérimentaux irradiés et non-irradiés." *Inst. de Rech. de Radiol. et de Radio-Hygiène National* (Budapest 1975): 1–10.

Bordas, E. and M. Deleanu. "Influence of negative air ions on experimental ulcer induced by pylorus ligature in albino rat." *Med Interne* (Oct–Dec 1989): 27(4): 313–317.

David, T. A., Minehart, J. R., and I. H. Kornblueh. "Polarized air as an adjunct in the treatment of burns." *Amer Jour of Phys Med* (1960): 39: 111–113.

Deleanu, M. and E. Bordas. "Morphological changes of the hypophysis-adrenal system (HAS) in albino rats with experimental gastric ulcers, under the influence of aeroionotherapy (AIT)." *Rom J Intern Med* (Jul–Dec 1991): 29(3–4): 215–20.

Gualtierotti, R., Kornblueh, I. H., and C. Sirtori, eds. *Aeroionotherapy.* Milan: Carlo Erba Foundation, 1960.

Iwama, H., Ohmizo, H., et al. "Inspired superoxide anions attenuate blood lactate concentrations in postoperative patients." *Critical Care Medicine* (June 2002): 30(6): 1246–1249.

Jaskowski, J., Mysliwski, A., et al. "Effect of air ions on L 1210 cells: changes in fluorescence of membrane-bound 1,8-aniline-naphthalene-sulfonate (ANS) after in vitro exposure of cells to air ions." *General Physiology and Biophysics* (Oct 1986): 5(5): 511–515.

Kornbleuh, Igho, et al. "Polarized Air as an Adjunct in the Treatment of Burns." Philadelphia: Northeastern Hospital, 1959.

Mäkelä, P., Ojajärvi, J., Graeffe, G., and M. Lehtimäki. "Studies on the effects of ionization on bacterial aerosols in a burns and plastic surgery unit." *J Hyg (Lond)* (Oct 1979): 83(2): 199–206.

Takahashi, K., Otsuki, T., Mase, A., Kawado, T., Kotani, M., Ami, K., Matsushima, H., Nishimura, Y., Miura, Y., Murakami, S., Maeda, M., Hayashi, H., Kumagai, N., Shirahama, T., Yoshimatsu, M., and K. Morimoto. "Negatively-charged air conditions and responses of the human psycho-neuro-endocrino-immune network." *Environ Int* (Aug 2008): 34(6): 765–772.

Wakamura, T., Sato, M., Sato, A., Dohi, T., Ozaki, K., Asou, N., Hagata, S., and H. Tokura. "A preliminary study on influence of negative air ions generated from pajamas on core body temperature and salivary IgA during night sleep." *Int J Occup Med Environ Health* (2004): 17(2): 295–298.

Pain

Hawkins, L. H. "The influence of air ions, temperature and humidity on subjective wellbeing and comfort." *Journal of Environmental Psychology* (1981): 1(4): 279–292.

Jonassen, Neils. "Are Ions Good For You?" *In Compliance* (August 1, 2013): www.incompliancemag.com/article/are-ions-good-for-you.

Kornbleuh, Igho, et al. "Polarized Air as an Adjunct in the Treatment of Burns." Philadelphia: Northeastern Hospital, 1959.

Robert, Hervé. *Ionisation, santé, vitalité, ou, Les bienfaits des ions négatifs de l'air*. Edité par Artulen (1991).

Soyka, F. *The Ion Effect*. New York, NY: Bantum Premium, 1983.

Mood

Frey, A.H. "Human behavior and atmospheric ions." *Psychol Rev* (May 1961): 68: 225–228.

Frey, A.H. "Modification of the conditioned emotional response by treatment with small negative air ions." *J Comp Physiol Psychol* (Feb 1967): 63(1): 121–125.

Frick, A. et al. "Serotonin Synthesis and Reuptake in Social Anxiety Disorder: A Positron Emission Tomography Study." *JAMA Psychiatry* (2015): 72(8): 794–802.

Goel, N., Terman, M., Terman, J.S., Macchi, M.M., and J.W. Stewart. "Controlled trial of bright light and negative air ions for chronic depression." *Psychol Med* (2005): 35(7): 945–955.

Krueger, A.P. "Are negative ions good for you?" *New Scientist* (June 1973): 58(850): 668–670.

Krueger, A.P., Andrfese, P. C., and S. Kotaka. "Small air ions: their effect on blood levels of serotonin in terms of modem physical theory." *Int J Biometeor* (1968): 12: 225–239.

Krueger, A.P., Kotdca, S., Kogure, Y., Takenobou, M., P.C. Ardriese. "Air ion effects on the growth of the silkworm (Bombyx mari. L.)." *Int J Biometeor.* (1966): 10: 29–38.

Krueger, A.P. and S. Sfgel. "Ions in the air." *Human Nature* (July 1978): 1(7):46–52.

Krueger, A.P., Strubbe, A.E., Yogt, M.G., and E.J. Reed. "Electric fields, small air ions and biological effects." *Int J Biometeor* (1978): 22: 202–212.

Livanova, L.M., Levshina, I.P., Nozdracheva, L.V., Elbakidze, M.G., and M.G. Airapetiants. "The protective action of negative air ions in acute stress in rats with different typological behavioral characteristics." *Zh Vyssh Nerv Deiat Im I P Pavlova* (May–June 1998): 48(3): 554–557.

National Institute of Mental Health. www.nimh.nih.gov.

Perez, V., Alexander, D.D., and W.H. Bailey. "Air ions and mood outcomes: a review and meta-analysis." *BMC Psychiatry* (Jan 2013): 13: 29.

Pino, O. and F. La Ragione. "There's Something in the Air: Empirical Evidence for the Effects of Negative Air Ions (NAI) on Psychophysiological State and Performance." *Research in Psychology and Behavioral Sciences* (2013): 1(4): 48–53.

Sakakibara, K. "Influence of negative air ions on drivers." *Research Domain 17, Toyota Central R&D Labs, R&D Review of Toyota CRDL* (2002): 37(1).

Scutti, Susan. "Social Phobia Linked to High Levels of Serotonin: Time to Rethink SSRIs and Other Anxiety Drugs?" www.medicaldaily.com. June 17, 2015.

Terman, M. and J.S. Terman. "Controlled trial of naturalistic dawn simulation and negative air ionization for seasonal affective disorder." *Am J Psychiatry* (Dec 2006): 163(12): 2126–2133.

Terman, M. and J.S. Terman. "Treatment of seasonal affective disorder with a high-output negative ionizer." *J Altern Complement Med* (Jan 1995): 1(1): 87–92.

Terman, M., Terman, J.S., and D.C. Ross. "A controlled trial of timed bright light and negative air ionization for treatment of winter depression." *Arch Gen Psychiatry* (Oct 1998): 55(10): 875–882.

Ucha Udabe, R., Kertész, R., and L. Franceschetti. "Études sur l'utilisation des ions négatifs dans les maladies du système nerveux." *Bioclimatology, Biometeorology and Aeroionotherapy.* Gualtierotti, R., Kornblueh, I. H., and C. Sirtori, eds. Milano: Carlo Erba Foundation, 1968: 128–134.

Watanabe, I. and Y. Mano. "Immunological Effect of Long-term Exposure of Negative Air Ions on Human." *The Journal of the Japanese Society of Balneology, Climatology and Physical Medicine.* (2000–2001): 64(3): 121; (2000–2001): 64(3): 123–128.

Cognitive Performance

Assael, M., Pfeifer, Y., and F. G. Sulman. "Influence of artificial air ionisation on the human electroencephalogram." *International Journal of Biometeorolog* (Dec 1974): 18(4): 306–312.

Baron, R.A. "Effects of negative ions on cognitive performance." *J Appl Psychol* (Feb 1987): 72(1): 131–137.

Duffee, R. A. and R.H. Koontz. "Behavioral effects of ionized air on rats." *Pyschophysiology* (1965): 1: 347–359.

Hawkins, L.H. and T. Barker. "Air ions and human performance." *Ergonomics* (Apr 1978): 21(4): 273–278.

Minkh, A. A. "The Effect of Ionized Air on Work Capacity and Vitamin Metabolism." *Journal of the Academy of Medical Sciences, U.S.S.R.* (1961): Translated by U.S. Department of Commerce, Washington, D.C.

Sakakibara, K. "Influence of negative air ions on drivers." *Research Domain 17, Toyota Central R&D Labs, R&D Review of Toyota CRDL* (2002): 37(1).

Soyka, F. and A. Edmonds. *The Ion Effect.* New York, NY: Dutton & Co. Publ., 1977.

Straus. H., Deleanu, M., and E. Florea. "Improvement of results of training in athletes under the influence of moderate negative aeroionization." *Med Sport (Roma)* (Mar 1965): 59: 171–175.

Sulman, F.G. *Health, Weather and Climate.* Basel, Switzerland: Karger, 1976.

Athletic Performance

Minkh, A. A. "The Effect of Ionized Air on Work Capacity and Vitamin Metabolism." *Journal of the Academy of Medical Sciences, U.S.S.R.* (1961): Translated by U.S. Department of Commerce, Washington, D.C.

Straus. H., Deleanu, M., and E. Florea. "Improvement of results of training in athletes under the influence of moderate negative aeroionization." *Med Sport (Roma)* (Mar 1965): 59: 171–175.

Cardiovascular Health

Deleanu, M. and M. Mozes-lörincz. "Effect of negative air ion exposure on adaptation to physical effort in young sportsmen." *Biometeorology* (1975): 6(I). Landsberg, H. E. and S. W. Tromp, eds. *Int J Biometeor Supplement* Vol. 19: 131.

Freed, C.R., Echizen, H., and D. Bhaskaran. "Brain serotonin and blood pressure regulation: studies using in vivo electrochemistry and direct tissue assay." *Life Sci* (Nov 1985): 37(19): 1783–1793.

Portnov, F. G. *Electroaerosol Therapy.* Zinatne, Riga, 1976.

Straus. H., Deleanu, M., and E. Florea. "Improvement of results of training in athletes under the influence of moderate negative aeroionization." *Med Sport (Roma)* (Mar 1965): 59: 171–175.

Yamada, S. and D. Chino. "Inhibitory effects of NAI on erythrocyte aggregation." *Med & Biology* (2000): 141(3): 79–83.

Free Radicals

Kosenko, E.A., Kaminsky, Yu. G., Stavrovskaya, I.G., Sirota, T.V., and M.N. Kondrashova. "The stimulatory effect of negative air ions and hydrogen peroxide on the activity of superoxide dismutase." *FEBS Lett* (June 1997): 410(2–3): 309–312.

Serotonin Irritation Syndrome (SIS)

Diamond, M. *Enriching Heredity: The Impact of the Environment on the Anatomy of the Brain.* New York, NY: Free Press, 1988.

Diamond, M.C. et al. "Environmental influence on serotonin and cyclic nucleotides in rat cerebral cortex." *Science* (1980): 210: 652–654.

Krueger, A. P., Andriese, P. C., and S. Kotaka. "Small air ions: Their effect on blood levels of serotonin in terms of modern physical theory." *International Journal of Biometeorology* (July 1968): 12(3): 225–239.

Krueger, A.P. and D.S. Sobel. *Air Ions and Health.* New York, NY: Harcourt Brace Jovanovich Inc., 1979.

Sulman, F.G. "Migraine and headache due to weather and allied causes and its specific treatment." *Ups J Med Sci Suppl* (1980): 31: 41–44.

Sulman, F.G., Levy, D., Lunkan, L., Pfeifer, Y., and E. Tal. "New methods in the treatment of weather sensitivity." [Article in German] *Fortschr Med* (Mar 1977): 95(11): 746–752.

Yates, A., Gray, F.B., Misiaszek, J.I., and W. Wolman. "Air ions: past problems and future directions." *Environment International* (1986): 12: 99–108.

Sleep

Misiaszek, J., Gray, F., and A. Yates. "The calming effects of negative air ions on manic patients: a pilot study." *Biol Psychiatry* (Jan 1987): 22(1): 107–110.

Reilly, T. and I.C. Stevenson. "An investigation of the effects of negative air ions on responses to submaximal exercise at different times of day." *J Hum Ergol* (Tokyo) (Jun 1993): 22(1): 1–9.

Soyka, F. *The Ion Effect.* New York, NY: Bantum Premium, 1983.

CHAPTER 4

Inoué, S. and M. Kabaya. "Biological activities caused by far-infrared radiation." *Int J Biometeorol* (Oct 1989): 33(3): 145–150.

Meng, J., Jin, W., Liang, J., Ding, Y., Gan, K., and Y. Yuan. "Effects of particle size on far infrared emission properties of tourmaline superfine powders." *J Nanosci Nanotechnol* (Mar 2010): 10(3): 2083–2087.

"Ozone Generators That Are Sold As Air Cleaners." *United States Environmental Protection Agency (EPA)*. www.epa.gov/iaq/pubs/ozonegen.html#how_is_ozone_harmful.

Tully, Lisa. "Official Measures of Negative Ion Emissions of Sports Bands." *Energy Medicine Research Institute* (July 16, 2013).

Vatansever, F. and M.R. Hamblin. "Far infrared radiation (FIR): its biological effects and medical applications." *Photonics Lasers Med* (Nov 2012): 4: 255–266.

Yu, S.Y., Chiu, J.H., Yang, S.D., Hsu, Y.C., Lui, W.Y., and C.W. Wu. "Biological effect of far-infrared therapy on increasing skin microcirculation in rats." *Photodermatol Photoimmunol Photomed* (Apr 2006): 22(2): 78–86.

About the Author

Earl Mindell, RPh, MH, PhD, is a registered pharmacist, college educator, and internationally recognized expert on nutrition, drugs, vitamins, and herbal remedies. He is also an award-winning author of over twenty best-selling books, including *Earl Mindell's New Vitamin Bible.* Dr. Mindell was inducted into the California Pharmacists Association's Hall of Fame in 2007. He was given the President's Award from the National Nutritional Food Association for his longtime contributions to the natural products industry in 2002, and was awarded the President's Citation for Exemplary Service from Bastyr University in 2012.

Dr. Mindell is on the Board of Directors of the California College of Natural Medicine and serves on the Dean's Professional Advisory Group, School of Pharmacy, Chapman University. He has appeared on numerous radio programs and television shows, including *The Oprah Winfrey Show, Live with Regis and Kathie Lee,* and *Good Morning America.*

Index

F

G

H

I

K

M

N

O

P

S

T

U

V

W

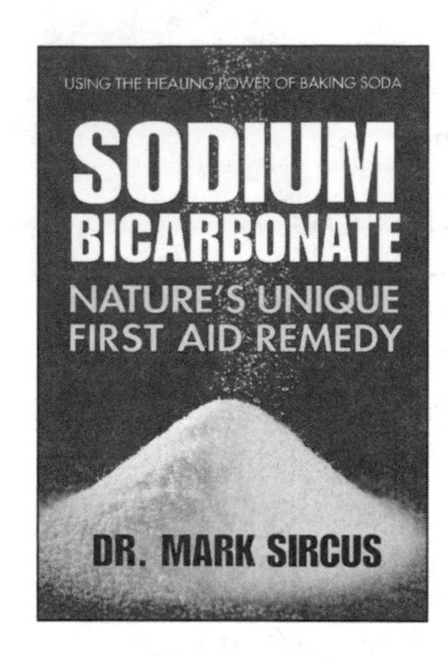

Sodium Bicarbonate

Nature's Unique First Aid Remedy

Dr. Mark Sircus

What if there were a natural health-promoting substance that was inexpensive, available at any grocery store in the country, and probably sitting in your cupboard right now? There is. It is called sodium bicarbonate, although you may know it as baking soda. For years, sodium bicarbonate has been used on a daily basis as part of a number of hospital treatments, but most people remain unaware of its full therapeutic potential. In his new book, Dr. Mark Sircus shows how this common compound along with magnesium, potassium, and calcium bicarbonates, may be used in the alleviation, or possibly even prevention, of many forms of illness.

Sodium Bicarbonate begins with a basic overview of the everyday item known as baking soda, chronicling its long history of use as an effective home remedy. It then explains the role sodium bicarbonate plays in achieving optimal pH balance, which is revealed as an important factor in maintaining good health. The book goes on to detail how sodium bicarbonate and its effect on pH may benefit sufferers of a number of conditions, including kidney disease, fungal infection, colds and flu, periodontal disease, hypertension, and even cancer, as well as its role in treating radioactive, chemical, and heavy metal toxicity. Finally, it lists the various ways in which sodium bicarbonate may be taken, suggesting the easiest and most effective method for your situation.

By providing a modern approach to this time-honored remedy, *Sodium Bicarbonate* illustrates the need to see baking soda in a whole new light. While it was once considered simply an ingredient in baked goods and toothpaste, sodium bicarbonate contains powerful properties that may help you balance your system, regain your well-being, and avoid future health problems.

$16.95 • 208 pages • 6 x 9-inch quality paperback • ISBN 978-0-7570-0394-3

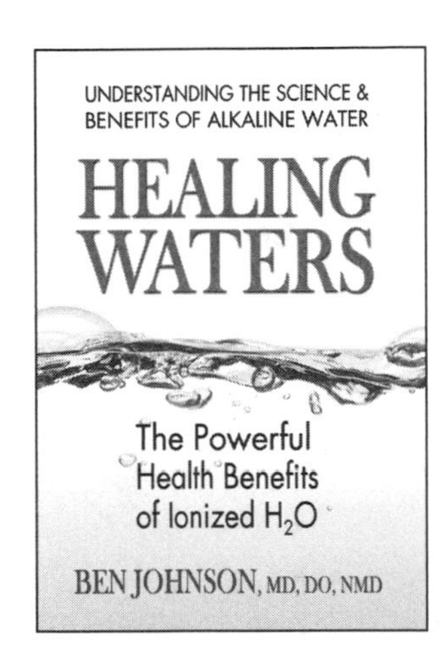

HEALING WATERS

The Powerful Health Benefits of Ionized H_2O

Ben Johnson, MD, DO, NMD

Acid-alkaline balance is the key to optimum health, and now you can achieve it simply by drinking nature's most bountiful liquid—water. In this revolutionary book, Dr. Ben Johnson guides you to oxygen-rich ionized water, H_2O that has been altered through the safe and simple process of electrolysis. Filled with antioxidants and alkalizing minerals, ionized water not only provides the body with a substance that is essential to all functions and life in general—water—but also restores the body's natural balance and maximizes well-being.

Healing Waters begins by explaining why water is crucial to good health. It then explores the importance of the body's acid-alkaline balance and examines why problems regarding this vital balance are responsible for many chronic conditions, including widespread problems such as diabetes and high blood pressure. Most importantly, the author reveals everything you need to know about ionized water, a natural remedy that is both pure and amazingly effective. You will learn how to buy, install, and use your own water ionizer so that your kitchen may be turned into a healthful oasis. You will discover that even the byproducts of the ionizing process may be used as a tool to enhance well-being. The author even provides nutritional tips for balancing your biological system easily and naturally.

The Fountain of Youth may be just another tall tale or legend, but with the power of *Healing Waters,* you will understand that a good source of health and longevity may be no farther than your very own home.

$15.95 • 128 pages • 6 x 9-inch quality paperback • ISBN 978-0-7570-0328-8

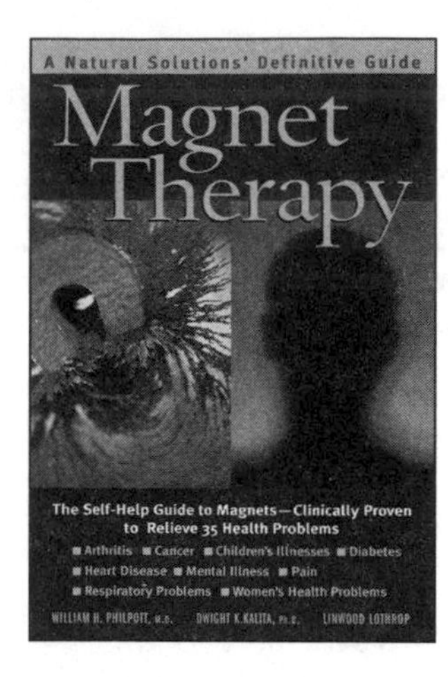

MAGNET THERAPY

SECOND EDITION

The Self-Help Guide to Magnets—Clinically Proven to Relieve 35 Health Problems

William H. Philpott, MD

Dwight K. Kalita, PhD

Linwood Lothrop

Remember when you were a kid and you raked a magnet through the sand, excited to find that when you took it out it was covered with specks of iron? Well, magnets work the exact same way on our bodies by manipulating the iron in our bloodstream. The magnets increase circulation, which then improves the way the body functions. The new edition of *Magnet Therapy* is filled with practical information as well as success stories that will bolster your determination to work toward greater health.

You would be amazed to learn just how many conditions can be healed with magnet therapy. Diabetes, heart disease, and multiple sclerosis are only three of the thirty-five health issues that this book discusses. Conventional medicine does its best with pills and other medications, but it treats only the symptoms. Alternative medicine, such as magnet therapy, seeks to treat the body as a whole so that your disorder is remedied through the enhancement of your well-being.

Whether this is your first time using magnets or your fortieth, *Magnet Therapy* will teach you to maximize your health in a way that is both scientifically proven and easy to understand.

$17.95 • 248 pages • 5.25 x 8.25-inch quality paperback • ISBN 978-0-7570-0332-5